Sleep-Related Female Orgasms

A Survey of Biological, Psychological, Sociological, and Cultural Factors

By

Franceen King, Ph.D.

 Self-Awareness Publishing Co.

A Division of The Self-Awareness Institute
Lutz, FL 33559

First revision: December, 2011
ISBN-13: 978-1468041828

Additional copies may be obtained from:
www.franceenking.com
www.amazon.com

Correspondence: DrFranceen@aol.com

AUTHOR'S NOTE

This book is a very slight revision of my 2006 Doctoral Dissertation, submitted to the faculty of the American Academy of Clinical Sexologists, then at Maimonides University, to fulfill requirements for the Ph.D. degree in Clinical Sexology. I decided to publish it in book form at this time (2011) because there seems to be a growing interest in **Sleep-Related Female Orgasms** (SRFOs), and there is currently very little information available to the general public.

The style of this book was designed to meet the requirements of my dissertation committee for a scholarly literature review. Therefore, it is rather academic and impersonal. Nonetheless, it covers a broad range of fascinating information, research data, and opinion about women's orgasms and sexuality. It is my hope that you will find it both interesting and helpful.

I will soon be publishing a companion book, **Waking Into the "Big O"** (2012), which is written in a more popular style, including more current statistical information, questions and answers, and commentary from women today who experience these SRFOs.

ACKNOWLEDGEMENTS

First and foremost I want to acknowledge Alfred C. Kinsey, whose passionate curiosity, commitment, and courage brought so many truths about human sexuality into the light of intelligent discussion. Without his work, almost nothing about this topic would be known.

I also acknowledge my many professional colleagues, clients, friends, workshop participants, and survey respondents who eagerly shared their stories with me, and repeatedly emphasized their opinions that this topic merits more research and public awareness.

I greatly appreciate the comments, editing, and sensitivity to language provided by my dissertation committee chairman,
Dr. Janice Epp, then Dean of Curriculum Development at the Institute for Advanced Study of Human Sexuality.

Lastly, I acknowledge my husband, Raymond Schmidt, who provided a wide range of household support and encouragement during the preparation of this paper, and my son, Robert Schmidt, who provided humor, computer assistance, and occasional proofreading.

ABOUT THE AUTHOR

As a Licensed Mental Health Counselor, Dr. Franceen King has had a clinical practice in Lutz, Florida, since 1981. Through her business, *The Self-Awareness Institute*, she has worked with individuals, couples, and groups in a counseling setting, and conducted workshops on a wide variety of topics throughout the state of Florida.

Since 1986, she has also designed and conducted week-long residential programs at *The Monroe Institute* in Virginia on topics related to consciousness expansion and exploration. She conducts outreach workshops throughout the world, especially Japan, using *TMI*'s Hemi-Sync© technology. Her life-long interests in lucid dreaming and paranormal perception have led her to explore many different philosophies and disciplines.

She began her career in the Washington, D.C. area where she spent seven years at the National Institutes of Health, first as a management intern and then as an employee development specialist, focusing on Executive Development and Organization Development. After leaving NIH, she formed a training and consulting firm, *Spectrum Associates, Inc.*, which provided services to numerous government agencies.

Her move to Florida in 1980, shifted the focus of her work from organizations to individuals. Since 1995, she has been an ordained minister in *Church of the Creator* with special interest in spiritual healing modalities.

She received her B.A. degree (psychology) from Mary Washington College of the University of Virginia (now Mary Washington University), her M.A. degree (community mental health counseling) from Hood College in Frederick, MD, and her Ph.D. (clinical sexology) from The American Academy of Clinical Sexologists, now in Winter Park, FL.

DEDICATION

This book is dedicated to all women,
in celebration of our bodies, minds, and Spirit!

TABLE OF CONTENTS

ABSTRACT

This study looks at the phenomenon of *sleep-related female orgasms* (SRFOs), often referred to as *female nocturnal orgasms.* This paper began with a simple question, "Why don't more people know that women can, and do, experience sleep-related orgasms?" Some of the answers have included 1) lack of inclusion in sex education classes; 2) lack of contemporary research; 3) lack of public discussion; and 4) historical association with powerful fear-based religious beliefs.

The study summarizes what is known about SRFOs based on existing research and historical opinion in fields of sexology, physiology, psychology, sleep, dreaming, anthropology and spirituality. While Kinsey noted that there is no single factor or cluster of factors that is predictive of SRFOs in an individual history, the strongest predictors in his research were frequent waking orgasm and "erotic responsiveness," low availability of other psycho-sexual outlets, masturbation, and fantasy during masturbation (Kinsey et al. 1953, 212-15). Today research suggests that overall, sleep mentations are more continuous than compensatory, and that sexual content and orgasmic experience during sleep are more likely among women who think about sex when awake. Waking cognitions include memory, fantasy, desire, imagination, prosexual attitudes, knowledge of SRFOs, and familiarity/safety with sexual pleasure and the orgasmic reflex. It is likely that formal education, intelligence, personality characteristics, and other cultural factors also influence these sleep mentations. Orgasmic responses during sleep seem more likely when there is some level of autonomic nervous system arousal before sleep, including both psychological and physiological elements. Physiological elements include lingering arousal from waking orgasms or other sexual behavior; however, this arousal may also be due to hormonal fluctuations, physical exercise, or emotional states such as anxiety, or anger. In these latter cases, SRFOs might serve a compensatory role in maintaining system homeostasis. It is likely that SRFOs occur more frequently among lucid dreamers due to possible neurological conditions unique to the lucid dream state, and the conscious freedom to exercise volition by choosing pleasure. SRFOs appear to be neither unhealthy nor rare.

Findings of the study suggest that the term *female nocturnal orgasms* needs to be replaced with the term *Sleep-Related Female Orgasms,* which is a more accurate designation of the phenomenon since these occurrences are diurnal as well as nocturnal. Additionally, the researcher lists twenty-seven possible hypotheses based on an extensive literature review that could be used in future research on the topic, and recommends that the topic be included in sex education classes for adolescents and continuing education modules for heath care professionals.

INTRODUCTION

Erotic dreams among women have been documented since the early Greek civilization; however, only in the past one hundred years have researchers begun to study the incidence and dynamics of sleep-related female *orgasms* (Kinsey et al. 1953, 191). While it is widely known that most men occasionally experience *wet dreams,* it appears that many adults in contemporary American culture are unaware that many women experience sleep-related orgasms. Given the prevalence of these responses (37 percent of women by age forty-five in Kinsey et al. 1953, and likely higher now), this lack of awareness is somewhat surprising. Realistically, however, this topic is rarely discussed. In addition, as will be shown, *the dynamics and etiology of these female sleep-related orgasms are somewhat different than the nocturnal emissions of men.*

Interest in this topic began while testing sample survey questions for a different topic. The issue of female sleep and dream-related orgasms kept surfacing. Two respondents reported that they mentioned these occurrences to their male therapists only to be told that the therapists had "never heard of such a thing." Subsequent inquiries have revealed that this is not unusual. An informal survey by this writer suggests that in 2005, approximately 70 percent of men did not know that women can experience sleep-related orgasms. It is even more surprising that a significant percentage of women, in excess of 25 percent, lacked this information.

Informal inquiries also suggest that women, who *do* experience sleep-related orgasms, enjoy them. This writer recently spoke to a mixed-sex group, ages twenties through sixties, and mentioned that while Kinsey found that the active incidence of female sleep-related orgasms peaked in the forty and fifty age decades, the accumulated incidence continued to increase throughout the lifespan (Kinsey et al. 1953). The women in the group started cheering! Dream therapist Gayle Delaney reports that she has "never heard a woman tell about an orgasmic dream that was not pleasurable" (Delaney 1994, 26). Kinsey and others have also noted this favorable reaction.

Therefore, one question this paper will address is simply, "Why don't more people know that women can, and do, experience sleep-related orgasms?" Obviously, lack of education plays a role. Contemporary sex education classes teach boys "such terms as 'nocturnal emission' . . . without a parallel terminology for girls' own nighttime orgasm" (Sweeney 1999). Although Kinsey found that 5 percent of his female respondents experienced their first orgasm as a sleep-generated orgasm (Kinsey et al. 1953, 193), this topic is not included in recommended sex education curriculums of any organization reviewed by this author for inclusion at any age level (i.e., American Academy of Pediatrics, 2001, Sexuality Information and Education Council of the United States, 1996, Kempner [SIECUS] 2003). Likewise, it is not included in literature from common public sex education forums such as Planned Parenthood (www.plannedparenthood.org). Virtually all curriculums and information scurces include commentary regarding male nocturnal emissions. One might conclude that women typically learn about sleep-related female orgasms through experience, although this hypothesis has not been tested. And there still is no accurate, standardized terminology for this experience in the research or educational literature.

A common initial response to the above-mentioned question is that this is another example of how attention to women's health has been neglected by the culture and mainstream researchers. The field of sexology has not been immune from this charge, as pointed out by Janice Irvine in *Disorders of Desire: Sex and Gender in Modern American Sexology:*

> Scientific sexology responds to feminism by minimizing it. The "ignore it and it'll go away" approach characterizes an enormous cross-section of American sexology. This tactic, perhaps the most dangerous, is reflected in the virtual absence of feminist analysis and scholarship within sexual science . . . Structural aspects of sexology perpetuate male dominance and inhibit feminist intervention." (Irvine 1990, 144-5)

There has been almost no research regarding this topic since the groundbreaking study by Kinsey, Pomeroy, Martin, and Gebhard

5

(Kinsey et al. 1953), which will be explored in detail below. In 1970, Gebhard, Raboch, and Geise noted the lack of follow-up information regarding this topic; and more recently Dr. Arnall of the British Psychological Society called this a "shamefully under researched area" (in Martell 2003).

This topic lies clearly within the scope of sexology; yet, it interfaces and penetrates other fields of inquiry more deeply than many other sexological topics. While research is therefore more complex, it will ultimately provide greater sexological insight. In addition to the normal physiological, psychological, and cultural variables that relate to sexological research, the fields of sleep physiology, dreaming, consciousness, anthropology, and spirituality contribute to awareness and understanding of this phenomenon. The mind-body relationship comes to the forefront providing sharp contrast to the emphasis on "structural aspects of sexology" mentioned by Irvine above.

Yet, it would be misleading to attribute the lack of awareness of sleep-related female orgasms to research and educational neglect alone. This topic has commanded much attention during other periods of Western civilization. Unfortunately, as was the case for sleep, dreams, and sex in general, the attention was based largely on superstition, fear, and moral judgment. The most severe consequences came during the three hundred year witch-burning epoch, mandated by the 1486 publication of the Catholic Church-initiated document, the *Malleus Maleficarum* of Kramer and Sprenger (Stewart 2002, 17-19; Masters 1966).

By the late eighteenth and nineteenth centuries, the sexual discourse had shifted more fully back into the medical model, its domain during the Greek and Roman periods, prior to the Christian church (Foucault, 1978, 1985). While the nature of the moral judgments and physical punishments changed, sleep-related female orgasms, like spermatorrhea (male emissions) and masturbation, were nonetheless viewed as both psychologically and physiologically pathological (Tissot 1758, and others including Freud 1900) until the 1920s, when they were then thought to be biologically compensatory for lack of other satisfactory sexual outlets (Kinsey et al. 1953, 207). To a great extent, Kinsey's data dispelled the compensatory imperative as a primary causative factor, thus leaving confusion, mystery, and relative silence. The dominant theory since Kinsey's time could be called the *system maintenance* model (Reinisch 1990, 89), which implies a randomness not really supported by the meager information at hand.

As Charles Stewart of the Royal Anthropological Institute points out:

> Erotic dreams have raised perennial questions about the boundaries of the self and individual's ability to control and produce this self. Do erotic dreams result from divine intercession, an immoral life, or recent memories? Are they products of the self for which the individual dreamer may be held responsible? Or are they

determined by a force majeure such as original sin, or human physiology? (Stewart 2002, 2)

These questions and associated fears still exist today as evidenced by numerous internet blog comments. The current lack of intelligent discussion provides fertile ground for more fear and confusion. Nonetheless, one of the few surveys conducted since Kinsey suggests that the incidence of sleep-related female orgasms is increasing significantly, influenced strongly by attitudes, education, and other cultural factors (Wells 1986). While professional journals ignore this, the Internet blogs and advice columns do not.

This paper provides literature review research regarding Sleep-Related Female Orgasms (SRFOs) and factors associated with these responses, research regarding the dynamics of female sex dreams (which often precede SRFOs), the history of attitudes and cultural responses toward SRFOs, and possible reasons why knowledge of SRFOs is apparently withheld from both men and women. It will explore social, behavioral, physiological, psychological, spiritual, moral, and political factors that influence and relate to this response, and make recommendations regarding further research and educational initiatives.

CHAPTER 1: DEFINITIONS AND EXAMPLES

Sleep Related Female Orgasms (SRFOs)

Most technical terms used in this paper will be defined as they are encountered in the narrative. However, it is useful at this point to define the topic of the paper more clearly. As mentioned above, there is no standard, accurate terminology in use when referring to sleep-related female orgasms. While Kinsey (1953) used the term "nocturnal orgasm" in his narrative, his chapter title was "Nocturnal Sex Dreams," and his formal designation was "sex dreams with orgasm." However, even in Kinsey's research, dream awareness did not always precede the experience of orgasm.

The *Kinsey Institute New Report on Sex* states, "Some men and women have orgasms during sleep. For men past puberty, this is called a nocturnal emission (or wet dream); for women and for boys before puberty it is called a nocturnal orgasm" (Reinisch 1990, 77). While *female nocturnal orgasm* is the most frequently encountered designation in professional literature, it is inaccurate because these responses are also diurnal, occurring during daytime naps. This fact is widely recognized by women experientially, and mentioned by Kinsey in a footnote (Kinsey et al. 1953, 191).

These experiences are also called "sleep orgasms," "dream orgasms," "spontaneous orgasms," "unconscious orgasms," "compensatory orgasms," "nocturnal pollutions," and "female wet dreams." As will be shown, all of these designations are inherently inaccurate, based on current knowledge of the etiology of this response.

A 1986 study by Barbara Wells sought to define this response more rigorously for research purposes, based on the subjective experience. While she used the inaccurate designation of "female nocturnal orgasm," she defined the experience as "when sexual arousal occurs during sleep and *wakes* one to perceive the experience of orgasm" (Wells 1986, 425). She comments further that "*Waking* to, with, or from orgasm initiated during sleep seemed a necessary distinction to make for this type of survey research with women . . . [since] even employing the discovery of vaginal secretions as the indicator of nocturnal orgasm is inconclusive evidence that orgasm, or even sexual excitement, has occurred during sleep" (Wells 1986, 425).

The shift in awareness from sleep to wakefulness is an important factor in both identifying and understanding this response. Therefore, the designation "awakening orgasms" would be accurate and useful if it did not carry so many other connotations. For purposes of this paper, the phrase "Sleep-Related Female Orgasms" (SRFOs) will be used as a generic reference to these awakening orgasms. Realistically, however, there are other categories of female orgasms that occur during sleep. These will be identified specifically as they are discussed.

Elements of Orgasm

Both Wells (1986) and Kinsey (1953) assumed that women were capable of determining for themselves whether or not orgasm had occurred. Nonetheless, it is useful for this discussion to review some of the currently recognized elements of orgasm.

Since 1966, the Masters and Johnson definition has been the primary physiological standard: "The outer third of the vagina . . . contracts strongly in a regularly recurring pattern . . . The contractions have onset at 0.8-second intervals and recur within a normal range of a minimum of three to five, up to a maximum of 10-15 times with each individual orgasmic experience" (Masters and Johnson 1966, 77-78). Masters and Johnson noted numerous other physiological elements which commonly occur, including contractions of the uterus and the anal and urethral sphincters, elevated heart rate and blood pressure, vasocongestion, skin flushing, and myotonia (Masters and Johnson 1966). Other researchers have noted increased pupil diameter (Wagner 1973), elevated pain thresholds (Whipple and Komisaruk 1985, 1988), a shift in brain laterality (Cohen et al. 1976), multiple changes in neurochemistry, significant deactivation of numerous brain structures (Holstege 2005a), and a wide variety of other physiological elements including increased electrical activity within the vagina (Shafik et al. 2004).

Helen Singer Kaplan emphasized that "the orgasm is, after all, a *reflex* [emphasis mine] and as such has a sensory and a motor component" (Kaplan 1974, 29). While researchers still debate the specific sensory and motor components, the reflexive nature of orgasm is very evident in SRFOs, especially when both genital stimulation and cognitive precursors are absent. Even when cognitive precursors (dreams) exist, the intensity of the orgasmic reflex is often a surprise. The physiology of SRFOs will be discussed in more detail in Chapter Three.

A recent paper on female orgasmic disorder includes the following comprehensive definition:

> Orgasm is a sensation of intense pleasure creating an altered consciousness state accompanied by pelvic striated circumvaginal musculature and uterine/anal contractions and myotonia that resolves sexually-induced vasocongestion and induces well-being/contentment. (Meston et al. 2004, 66)

For these massive physiological changes to be considered intensely pleasurable is ultimately a subjective interpretation/perception (Whipple et al. 1992, and others). A recent study suggests that for both men and women, "the subjective experience of orgasmic pleasure and satisfaction depends more on psychological and psychosocial than on physical factors" (Mah and Yitzchak 2005, 187). On the other hand, many of the physiological changes contribute directly to feelings of "well-being/ contentment."

For purposes of this paper, perhaps the most interesting part of the Meston et al. definition is the reference to orgasm as "creating an altered consciousness state" (Meston et al. 2004, 66). In the case of SRFOs, consciousness alters from sleep to wakefulness. Awareness often shifts from the bizarreness of a dream scenario to normal reality. Given that "dreaming is considered to be an altered state of consciousness . . . [and] lucid dreams can be considered an altered state of dreaming" (Van de Castle 1994, 444), there are multiple consciousness altering factors at play in the SRFO. This ability of orgasm to alter consciousness from a more expanded state to a more grounded, contracted state is important for many who spend extended periods of time in consciousness exploration. On the other hand, orgasm can also alter consciousness in the opposite direction.

It would be easy to argue that *all* stages of the human sexual response cycle alter consciousness, including the periods before, during, and after orgasm. In her groundbreaking book, *Transcendent Sex*, consciousness researcher Jenny Wade provides evidence that profoundly transcendent states of consciousness and experience do occur during all stages (Wade 2004). In the opinion of renowned consciousness researcher Ken Wilbur:

> That is why sex can kill you. As the simplest, most accessible, most here-and-now transcendent experience that anybody can have, it is the most common doorway to the Divine, the most ordinary (in the best sense of the word) altered state that accelerates the stages of

spiritual realization. The more one is plunged into the ocean of Spirit, into the ocean of infinite ease, the more one dies to one's smaller self, dies to one's ego, that finite and contracted and mortal coil, and finds instead one's own Original Face, one's own Godhead, one's own True Nature, prior to but not other to the entire manifest world. (Wilbur, in *Forward* to Wade 2004, xi)

The role of consciousness and psychological factors in SRFOs will be discussed more thoroughly in Chapters Five, Six, and Seven.

There is one other element of orgasm that merits attention in the exploration of SRFOs. That is the subjective experience of energy movement. Previous theories of SRFOs, as compensatory for lack of other sexual outlets, hypothesized an energy- balancing role; i.e., a discharge of excess or blocked sexual energy (Freud 1905; Reich 1942). The notion of *sexual* energy has lost favor in sexological research because, to date, there is no way to observe or quantify this energy. Nonetheless, the *experience* of energy movement, whether described as sexual energy or simply life energy, is well known to many, in both waking sex and SRFOs. The yogic traditions of the East acknowledge this energy movement in Tantric sex practices. As interpreted by sex therapist Judy Kuriansky, "Tantric sex redefines what sex is – not as an action, but as movement of energy within you individually, and between you and your partner. The practices guide you to generate sexual energy, transform it into love energy, and transmit it to your partner and even to the universe" (Kuriansky 2002, 24). Anecdotal reports, like those included in the next section,

14

suggest that both the cognitive precursors to SRFOs, and the after-effects, often include heightened energy awareness.

Examples of SRFOs

Due to the general lack of awareness regarding SRFOs, a few examples are included at this point to assure that the reader has some level of familiarity with the topic. While there appears to be a very wide range of possible SRFO experiences, the following kinds of reports are common. They will also provide reference points for future discussion.

Example #1: The first example is from this writer's personal experience, and took place quite recently. It is a classic example of an SRFO preceded by a simple, overtly sexual dream. It is interesting in that both the experience and the dream content took place on bright, sunny afternoons, thus highlighting the error of "nocturnal" as a designation.

> I was away from home, in the second week of a two-week business trip. I had an opportunity to take a nap following a late lunch. While sleeping, I became aware of a vivid, though not fully lucid, dream in which I was talking to a group of people on an outdoor pool deck adjacent to a large building like a hotel lobby. This felt like an informal reception or cocktail party. I was talking about my dissertation. One man in the group started talking to me. I could see him and hear him, but I could not comprehend what he was saying. So I moved closer to him and sat on a lounge chair next to him. At this point he moved on top of me and began sexual behavior. This surprised me, and I felt concerned about being in a

very public place. I then felt somewhat comforted by noticing a large potted plant shielding us from view. Contact with him felt very good and my body quickly began to orgasm both in the dream and physically.

This woke me up. I noticed that I could shift my awareness back and forth between normal waking awareness and the multi-sensory dream awareness. I could not, however, move the dream forward. It stopped during orgasm, at the point at which I was awakened. I stayed in bed for a while letting my body calm down, and reflecting on the experience. I noted that this occurred approximately 1 hour and 20 minutes into sleep . . . a normal time for REM stage sleep. I also noted that I had not been aware of any sexual feelings or intention prior to the nap or during the first part of the dream. The time between contact and orgasm seemed very brief, probably less than ten seconds.

Examples #2 and #3: These next examples come from Gayle Delaney's book *Sexual Dreams* (1994), and show how the dreams which proceed SRFOs are not always overtly sexual.

#2 - I was swimming with a dolphin in clear water. All I did was feel him rub along my belly and . . . Well, you get the picture. (Delaney 1994, 25)

#3 – I was on my childhood swing set teeter-totter. The experience became sexually arousing and ended with an outrageous nocturnal orgasm. (Delaney 1994, 26)

Example #4: This report shows the impact of lucidity, volition, and energy awareness. These factors will be discussed in Chapter Five.

> Briefly, all my sexual dreams that culminate in orgasm are lucid. The orgasms are quick, intense, full-body sensations and very pleasurable. The "Kundalini" [energy] begins to rise and I just go with the flow, sometimes with a partner whom I conjure up, sometimes with nobody. Sometimes I look around in the dream for some unsuspecting male whom I approach and seduce. (Delaney 1994, 26)

Example #5: Here is a typical report from a woman who learned about SRFOs by experience. Her initial reaction of concern is common.

> One month I was awakened by orgasms four or five different times. I have a good sex life with my husband, and I hardly ever masturbate, so I couldn't figure out why this was happening to me. I started to think that perhaps I was becoming a nymphomaniac, a person who could never get enough sexual satisfaction. Fortunately, I was able to discuss this with a woman who's a psychiatrist, and she set my mind at ease. (Masters, Johnson, and Kolodny 1982, 298)

Example #6: This report is from a pregnant on-line blogger. From Internet searches it would appear that SRFOs might be more common during pregnancy. There has been no research to verify this.

The last three nights in a row, I've had very vivid erotic dreams that end with me waking up and experiencing an intense orgasm. More intense even than those acquired through intercourse or other intimate means with [husband] or even through masturbation. Friday night's dream brought on such a powerful climax, that I had abdominal cramps for a few minutes, something I've been assured is normal and completely unharmful to the little peanut in my tummy . . . [An article I read] suggested that the person experiencing the 'wet dream' was fulfilling through sleep what they were neglected in their sex life. This is laughable to me, at least in my situation. (*The Good Wife* 2005)

Example #7: This question/report is from the WebMD advice column. It shows teen-age onset and possibly a compensatory pattern. More importantly, it reveals the writer's years of self-doubt and lack of terminology.

I was wondering if women can experience wet dreams. I have since I was in high school. As I got older and started to have sex they stopped, but now I notice that when I'm not getting sex very often I start having them again. It's really weird – I am extremely aroused in the dream, the dream only lasts for a few seconds, and I orgasm and wake up as it happens. It's the coolest thing. I mentioned it to my boyfriend some time ago, and he had never heard of it (but was very aroused by it!) I've never heard of this happening and am just wondering if I'm weird. (Weston 2005)

Example #8: Here is a similar question from an older woman. SRFOs can play a significant role in the lives of women who lack other satisfying social-sexual outlets.   This will be discussed further in Chapter Four.

> I would like to know the physiology aspects of "wet dreams" for women.   Even though I'm a 55-year-old woman, I admit there are many things I don't know or understand about my body.
>
> I haven't engaged in intercourse for more than five years, because   have no partner, but from time to time I enjoy the most intense nocturnal orgasms.   I wake up extremely aroused, sexually, and my clitoris and genitals very sensitive.   Yet I know I have not actually touched myself physically during the experience.
>
> These orgasms during sleep seem more intense than any I ever experience during intercourse and I have wondered how the thought and the brain can produce such a pleasant phenomenon.   P.S.   I do not dream of intercourse when this occurs. (Reinisch 1990, 88-89)

Example #9:   This last example comes from this writer's experience since no details of similar examples have been found in the literature.   It represents the soundtrack of one's thinking while waking into an orgasm that is *not* preceded by awareness of a dream, but only unconscious sleep.   It also demonstrates the experience of energy flow from expanded to more contracted.

> Yikes! What's happening? Where am I? O my God! I'm exploding into a million pieces.   Ahhhhhhhhhhhhhh. (Energy rushes, followed by jerk, jerk, jerk . . . dawning awareness of body) I think I have to pee. Man . . . I'm having an orgasm. . . . (contract, squeeze, contract, more energy sensations) Wow, this is intense! Oh my God!!! . .

    Wow! . . . . Whew! (Breathe, pant, pant, . . .
    giggle, giggle) . . . . That was fun!

This latter example is similar to dream researcher Patricia Garfield's comments about orgasms after she learned to become lucid in her dreams: "I began experiencing dream orgasms of profound intensity . . . I found myself bursting into soul- and body- shaking explosions" (Garfield 1979, 44). The role of dreams in SRFOs will be discussed further in Chapter Five.

CHAPTER 2: A REVIEW OF CONTEMPORARY SURVEY RESEARCH

The Kinsey Report

The contemporary history of SRFOs begins, and almost ends, with the Kinsey, Pomeroy, Martin, and Gebhard study of *Sexual Behavior in the Human Female* (Kinsey et al. 1953). While Kinsey used the term "nocturnal emissions" to describe the male experiences, his terminology for women was "sex dreams with orgasm" or "sex dreams without orgasm." Key results from this study are included at this point, since many of Kinsey's findings were truly revolutionary and play a pivotal role in our understanding; i.e., before Kinsey, after Kinsey. The basic data on this topic, as summarized by the Kinsey Institute, is as follows:

Nocturnal Sex Dreams and Orgasms:

Approximately two-thirds of females reported overtly sexual dreams (and Kinsey estimated over the life course that 70% of females experienced sex dreams), and almost 100% of the males (p.196, 215, *Female*).

By age 45, 37% of females in the sample had experienced a sex dream with orgasm (p. 196, *Female*); Kinsey reported that 83% of males reported nocturnal emissions, with or without dreams (p. 518-199, *Male*).

The frequencies with which the average female had nocturnal orgasms stayed fairly constant for single and married females of all ages (adolescence to 50 yrs. old), (p.200, *Female*). The highest incidence (70%) and frequency for males came in the late teens, but declined in the thirties, (p. 523, *Male*). (http://www.indian.edu/~kinsey/resources/ak-data.html)

This data for women was based on 5940 Caucasian females. Kinsey used two incidence measurements: *accumulated incidence* (occurrence at some point in lifetime), and *active incidence* (occurrence during past five years). In contrast to men, the highest *active incidences* of nocturnal orgasm for women overall occurred between ages forty and fifty-five. Comparing the *active incidences*,

> The peak for the single females had come at age forty with 22 per cent involved; it had come for the married females at age fifty with 32 percent involved. For the previously married females it had come at age fifty-five with 38 percent involved . . . Marital experience had evidently developed the imaginative capacities of some females who had not had sex dreams before marriage, and of a still larger number of those who had become widowed, separated or divorced. (Kinsey et al. 1953, 201)

Regarding the *accumulated incidence*, Kinsey noted that incidence of SRFOs was higher among married and previously married women than among never married women (Kinsey et al. 1953, 201). Kinsey attributed this to greater imagination. (This might suggest that memory and increased familiarity with the orgasmic reflex were also contributing factors.) Overall, "*the number of females who were dreaming to orgasm increased with advancing age*" (Kinsey et al. 1953, 201, emphasis mine). In addition, SRFOs provided a higher percentage of sexual outlet for older women than younger women, "as much as 14 per cent of the total outlet" for older, previously married women (Kinsey et al. 1953, 206).

While the *frequency* of SRFOs varied among individuals, and fluctuated greatly throughout any individual woman's life, overall, "the average frequencies for those who were having [orgasmic] dreams . . . remained around 3 to 4 times per year from adolescence to the oldest age groups . . . at least to age sixty-five"(Kinsey et al. 1953, 201). These frequencies were much more stable and well below the median male frequency of ten times per year at younger ages and five times per year when older (Kinsey et al. 1953, 668).

Among this sample, Kinsey also noted that the beginning of SRFOs, for ten percent of those who experienced them, occurred in the same year as the beginning of other types of sexual activity: masturbation, petting, coitus, or homosexual contact (Kinsey et al. 1953, 210). Ninety-five per cent of the women had experienced orgasm while awake before experiencing SRFOs, meaning, obviously, that "there are some females (5 per cent) . . . who experience nocturnal dreams to orgasm before they have ever experienced orgasm from any other source while they are awake" (Kinsey et al. 1953, 193). A very small, unspecified percentage of Kinsey's sample began experiencing SRFOs before age 10 (Kinsey et al. 1953, 197). By contrast 22 percent of the men in Kinsey's sample experienced their first ejaculation as a nocturnal emission (Kinsey, Pomeroy, and Martin 1948).

In addition, "there were some females, including as many as 2 per cent of those with masturbation in their histories, who were capable of reaching orgasm through fantasy alone" (Kinsey et al. 1953, 200). Kinsey noted that among both females and males, nocturnal sex dreams, more than any other type of sexual outlet, appear to have their origins in what are primarily psychologic stimuli" (Kinsey et al. 1953, 193).

Kinsey's data charts clearly indicate that women with higher social class upbringings reported more SRFOs (Kinsey et al. 1953, 219). The *accumulated incidence* was higher for upper level "parental occupational class" in every age range. Kinsey's narrative attributed this to "vagaries of sampling" (Kinsey et al. 1953, 203), rather than a significant trend.

Likewise, Kinsey's data charts clearly indicate that women with higher educational levels, especially graduate school, reported more SRFOs (Kinsey et al. 1953, 218). Among single women, the *active incidence* was highest for women with "17+" years of education in every age range, with *only* this educational group reporting active incidence in the age ranges above forty. For married and previously married women, the *active incidence* was highest for women with "17+" years of education in almost all age ranges. Perhaps something was lost in the averaging, however,

24

because Kinsey's narrative states "there seems to have been no correlation between the educational background of the female and the accumulative or active incidence of her nocturnal sex dreams . . . or the frequency with which she had such dreams to the point of orgasm" (Kinsey et al. 1953, 201). Nonetheless, several others have noted this discrepancy (Geddes 1954, 52; Tiefer 1995). It is also interesting to note that women who chose higher education, started experiencing SRFOs somewhat more often at younger ages (Kinsey et al. 1953, 218); and SRFOs provide a higher percentage of sexual outlet for highly educated women at all age levels, especially above age 35 (Kinsey et al. 1953, 563).

Kinsey does acknowledge these differences in his survey of men. He states, for example, "There are 10 to 12 times as frequent nocturnal emissions among males of the upper educational classes as there are among males of the lower classes" (Kinsey, Pomeroy, and Martin 1948, 345). "It is particularly interesting to find that there are [great] differences between educational levels in regard to nocturnal emissions – a type of sexual outlet which one might suppose would represent involuntary behavior" (Kinsey, Pomeroy, and Martin 1948, 343).

Regarding religiosity, Kinsey found that "fewer of the females who were active or devout religiously had dreamed to the point of orgasm – perhaps because they had had the smallest amount of overt sexual experience about which they could dream. On the other hand, the frequencies with which the females had had dreams after they had once started them did not seem to be affected by the religious background" (Kinsey et al. 1953, 205).

Overall, Kinsey considered masturbation and the frequency of orgasm derived through nocturnal dreams as "the activities which provide the best measure of a woman's intrinsic sexuality," since so many other sexual outlets depend on the presence of other persons (Kinsey et al. 1953, 192).

Kinsey also inquired about the content of sexual dreams preceding orgasm. In his sample, only one percent reported SRFOs without dreams (Kinsey et al. 1953, 212). The role of dreams will be explored in Chapter Five.

For historical context, one of the most important parts of Kinsey's report is his very thoughtful discussion of the "moral significance of nocturnal sex dreams" (Kinsey et al. 1953, 207-214). In order to address this thoroughly, Kinsey included a full sample of 7789 women in his discussions regarding morality and possible causal correlations. This included both white and "Negro" women, and both prison and non-prison cases (Kinsey et al. 1953, 208).

A popular thought at that time, coming out of the biologic/medical model, was that SRFOs represented a "natural" way for the body to compensate for the lack of sexual activity among those who voluntarily abstain. Therefore, "the frequencies of the dreams are supposed to have an inverse relation to the frequencies of other sexual activities, thus providing a safety valve for the 'sexual energy' which accumulates when other outlets are unavailable or are not being utilized" (Kinsey et al. 1953, 207). Several researchers before Kinsey addressed this topic. Regarding women specifically, Hammer asserted "that the female who is deprived of other sexual outlets will find relief in nocturnal orgasms once every third day. Mantegazza, however, says once in four or five days." (reported in Kinsey et al. 1953, 208). These writers did not present data to support their statements, and Kinsey's frequency data was much ower than these estimates.

This *compensatory* theory had been popularized since the beginning of the twentieth century, resulting in both Catholic and Jewish codes recognizing nocturnal dreams as "the only acceptable form of sexual outlet . . . outside of vaginal coitus," and then, only under strict conditions (Kinsey et al. 1953, 207).

Therefore, it was probably surprising to many that Kinsey's data did not strongly support the compensatory theory either in frequency or circumstance (Kinsey et al. 1953, 211). Only fourteen percent of his cases demonstrated any compensatory relationship whatsoever, and only under extreme circumstances; i.e., prison, or loss of a spouse. Even in those cases, the numbers of SRFOs were not nearly adequate to compensate for the loss of other outlets. If Kinsey had not included the prison population in his analysis, the rate of compensatory relationship would have been even lower. (The compensatory theory will be discussed further in Chapter Four, which addresses loss of sexual outlets, and Chapter Seven, which addresses spiritual, religious and moral issues related to SRFOs.)

On the other hand, seven percent of those who experienced SRFOs reported that they occurred most often during periods when they were actively involved in adequate or high rates of other sexual activity.   In addition, 89 percent of those who experienced the highest incidences of nocturnal orgasms (seventy-four women reported SRFOs at least once a week for at least five years) also experienced 100 percent orgasmic response during "coitus," and high rates of multiple orgasms (Kinsey et al. 1953, 210).

So if biologic compensation was not the main cause of SRFOs for Kinsey's sample, what was? He found a slight positive correlation between the occurrence of masturbation, and the occurrence of fantasies in masturbation with nocturnal orgasms (Kinsey et al. 1953, 211).   But overall Kinsey noticed that both physiological and psychological factors could operate in *different* ways at *different* times for even the same subjects. He concluded, "that no single factor or small group of factors may account for [SRFOs'] occurrence or non-occurrence in a history" (Kinsey et al. 1953, 212).

Realistically, there are a number of *physiological* factors related to SRFOs that Kinsey's study did not address. Chief among these would be the role of hormones during the monthly menstrual cycle, pregnancy, and menopause.   Illness and other physical conditions were not explored. And obviously, a wide variety of specific *psychological* factors could have an influence. Nonetheless, Kinsey's study provided far more information than had been previously available, and dispelled several myths.

It also raised some troubling questions. Since biological compensation was not a strong factor in the occurrence of sleep-related orgasms, how should these events be viewed morally? Since so many different factors might be influencing this response, where would future researchers begin their search for understanding? Both of these points have probably deterred many from pursuing further research.

Elements of the Kinsey data will be explored in more detail in some of the following chapters.

Survey Research Since Kinsey

In the years since Kinsey, there have been several large surveys of sexual behavior in the United States. None of these surveys have included questions or discussion related to SRFOs. Specifically, this topic was not included in *The Hite Report* (1976), *The Janus Report* (1993), or the University of Chicago National Health and Social Life Survey (NHSLS) (Laumann et al. 1994; Michael et al. 1994).

There have been only four formal survey studies related to SRFOs published since Kinsey's groundbreaking report. The most recent of these is twenty years old (Wells 1986). All suffer from extremely limited sample populations. Beyond these, there are simply anecdotal reports scattered throughout the literature and popular press. *No formal survey of SRFOs in healthy women over college age has been published since the Kinsey report.*

The first two post-Kinsey studies are interesting from a historical perspective because they reflect old notions about mental health as well as female sexuality. Both were conducted with patients from medical and surgical clinics and compared the incidence of reported SRFOs between women diagnosed as mentally ill and control groups of patients. In the first study, Tapia, Werboff, and Winokur (1958), it was "found that 47% of 59 women with the diagnosis of a neurosis reported nocturnal orgasm experience as opposed to 8% of the controls. In a replication study, Winokur, Guze, and Pfeiffer (1959) ascertained that 42% of 50 women with a diagnosis of psychosis, 46% of 50 women with a diagnosis of neurosis, and 6 % of 100 female controls reported the experience of nocturnal orgasms" (as reported in Wells 1986, 422).

Original copies of these studies were not available. However, given the lack of distinct categories of mental illness, and the fact that the control groups were also patient populations, it is difficult to assess these results. It can be noted, however, that among some medical practitioners in the early twentieth century, SRFOs were viewed *prima facie* as an indicator of neurosis. Some who held this opinion, according to Kinsey, included Kisch, Krafft-Ebing, Loewenfeld, and Bloch. Kinsey commented on this point:

> At various points in the literature the opinion has been expressed that nocturnal dreams in the female are an expression of some neurotic disturbance, and that "normal," well adjusted females do not dream to the point of orgasm. The very fact that nocturnal sex dreams are not as universal in the female as they are in the male seems to have contributed to the opinion that they are pathologic. There is a tendency to consider anything in human behavior that is unusual, not well known, or not well understood, as neurotic, psychopathic, immature, perverse, or an expression of some other sort of psychologic disturbance. Curiously enough, the persons who contend that sex dreams represent neurotic disturbances in the female admit that it is impossible to believe that 80 per cent or more of the male population is to be considered neurotic simply because that percentage has nocturnal sex dreams which effect orgasm. (Kinsey et al. 1953, 195)

This is one topic where women obviously owe Dr. Kinsey a debt of gratitude. (As will be discussed in Chapter Six, some modern personality theorists view SRFOs as indicators of high self-esteem, self-confidence, and creativity.)

The other two published research studies since Kinsey involved college-aged populations. Therefore, the incidence peaks in the age 40 and 50 decades, which surfaced in Kinsey's study, could not be observed.

In Henton (1976), 774 female African-American undergraduates were surveyed. Twenty-two percent reported the experience of nocturnal orgasm. In Wells (1986), 245 female undergraduate and graduate students (90 percent Caucasian) were surveyed. Thirty-seven percent reported the experience of nocturnal orgasm. Kinsey's data for women at age twenty indicated 8 percent reported nocturnal orgasms. If these three studies are comparable at all, they indicate a rapidly increasing incidence of SRFOs over the period of 1953 to 1986, a period which spans the sexual revolution in American culture. Moreover, since the 1976 and 1986 studies included only college women, it might suggest that level of formal education truly is a significant factor in the experience of SRFOs.

Despite its limited sample population, the Wells study was quite comprehensive and well designed. First of all, it specified a designation (female nocturnal orgasm), and defined the experience as *"when sexual arousal occurs during sleep and wakes one to perceive the experience of orgasm"* (Wells 1986, 425). It did not specifically define orgasm, but assumed, as did Kinsey, that "whether or not [the women] reach orgasm in these dreams is a matter about which few of them have any doubt" (Kinsey et al. 1953, 192). Kinsey also reported that "the female is often awakened by the muscular spasms or convulsions which follow her orgasms" (Kinsey et al. 1953, 192).

The Wells study used nine self-report, randomly-ordered, scales and inventories. It tested nine hypotheses, and assessed fifty-eight predictor variables. The volunteer subjects were told simply that they were participating in a study of "various facets of human sexuality." Before summarizing these results, it is interesting to note that "35% of this college sample reported they had never previously heard of nocturnal orgasms" (Wells 1983,1986).

Of the subjects who reported SRFOs, the average age of onset was 17.63; the average age of this sample population was 22.14. While the *incidence* of reported occurrences was much higher for this age group than the Kinsey study, the *frequency* of reported occurrences was only slightly higher – between four and five times per year.

A complex multivariate regression analysis of the fifty-eight variables revealed that very few of them had any predictive value. Some factors which were rejected in this regard included: sexual experiences, variety of sexual experiences, frequency of participation in seventeen different sexual activities, age, marital status, religiosity, frequency of sexual dreams.

Factors which were correlated with SRFOs included: satisfaction with one's sex life, high levels of erotic responsiveness (arousal), anxiety, *sexual liberalism, waking sexually excited from sleep, being familiar with the phenomenon of nocturnal orgasms, and/or having a positive attitude toward nocturnal orgasms.* The italicized items had the strongest predictive value. Anxiety was correlated with SRFOs in the Henton (1976) and Winokur, Guze, and Pfeiffer (1959) studies also, and will be discussed in Chapter Six.

Level of education was not a studied variable, yet obviously, was a common element in the sample population, and may itself have predictive value. While being familiar with the phenomenon of SRFOs was predictive, it describes a "chicken or the egg" kind of situation. Do women know about SRFOs and then experience them? Or do they become aware of SRFOs by experiencing them? The study participants were not asked how they became aware of SRFOs. It is likely that to date, women have become aware of SRFOs primarily by experiencing them. Both of these questions beg to be explored in future surveys.

Wells discusses the role of awareness and asks,

> Does knowledge of female nocturnal orgasms precede their occurrence or vice versa? If knowledge is the precedent, the consideration of the role of "power of suggestion " in this type of sleep behavior is interesting . . . Then too, a significant predictor of nocturnal orgasm experience is agreeing that, "most women have nocturnal orgasms." Perhaps those respondents with reported nocturnal orgasm experience have rationalized that their behavior fits into the "norm," even though research to this point indicates that the majority of women have not reported the experience of nocturnal orgasm. The respondents with experiences of nocturnal orgasm in the past year further removed themselves from deviant labels and association with abnormalities by disagreeing with the notion that this phenomenon is a reflection of neurotic tendencies. (Wells 1986, 435)

To a lesser degree, the issue of sexual liberalism poses the same question - which comes first? And given the cultural emphasis on sexual conservatism in the past twenty years, particularly in regard to sex education (Kempner [SIECUS] 2003), as well as fear of HIV and STDs, one might wonder if SRFOs are actually decreasing. In any event, the Wells study clearly suggests that cultural factors, as well as physiological and psychological indicators, affect the incidence of SRFOs. The role of these factors, and others, will be explored in the following chapters.

Other Sources of Information

Before leaving this discussion of survey research, it is useful to mention a small survey by on-line advice columnist Marcy Jarvis (2003). She became very frustrated when she could not find current information about SRFOs, and decided to survey women she knew, ages 22 to 38. "Thirteen out of 30 women [43%] admitted nocturnal orgasms, and the ages where they had first achieved them ranged from 16 to 27" (Jarvis 2003, 3). She had personally experienced her first orgasm through dreaming. As small as this survey is, other advice columnists cite it.

The most common sources of information for women today regarding SRFOs are advice columns in popular women's magazines (primarily *Cosmopolitan*, and *Redbook*), on-line advice columns, and a few Internet blogs.   Occasionally advice columns in men's magazines entertain questions related to SRFOs.   The typical question is some variation of example #7 in Chapter One: "Is it possible for women to have *wet dreams* or orgasms in their sleep?" followed by commentary about the inquirer's experience. Typically, the responses are brief; cite Kinsey's data; and then offer a wide range of accurate and/or inaccurate information.

Chapter 3: THE PHYSIOLOGY OF SLEEP-RELATED FEMALE ORGASMS

Many details about the physiology of SRFOs are simply unknown at this point in time. However, pieces of relevant information do exist which allow some degree of understanding or conjecture. Since SRFOs occur during sleep, a basic understanding of the human sleep cycle provides a useful starting point.

The Human Sleep Cycle

While knowledge of human sleep and sleep disorders continues to expand and change, the following description represents a basic summary of current understandings regarding the human sleep cycle. Prior to the 1950s, researchers thought that sleep was a passive, dormant, uniform condition. Since then, it has been discovered that human brains are extremely active during sleep, demonstrating differentiated phases and stages, and exhibiting up to five times more electrical activity than during wakefulness (Dement 1974). During normal sleep, human brain waves move through a typical pattern lasting approximately ninety minutes. This pattern or cycle is repeated throughout the night. It consists of two primary parts.

The first part, called the Non-Rapid Eye Movement (NREM) phase, consists of four stages. This is the orthodox, anabolic, physically-regenerating part of sleep, with stages three and four also

37

known as the slow-wave cycle. Stage three & four NREM sleep is characterized by very low frequency delta brain waves and can last as long as thirty or forty minutes per cycle (Flanagan 2000, 75), with longer periods toward the beginning of the night and shorter periods toward morning. "Unresponsiveness to environmental stimuli is most extreme during slow-wave sleep, whereas inertia or muscular activity is not" (Richardson 1966, 75). For example, sleep-walking, night terrors, bed-wetting, and other physical movements occur during NREM sleep even though the sleeper is totally unaware. This phase "coincides with the release of growth hormone in children and young adults. Many of the body's cells also show increased production and reduced breakdown of proteins during deep sleep . . . Activity in parts of the brain that control emotions, decision-making processes, and social interactions is drastically reduced during deep sleep" (NINDS 2005, 5).

The second part of the cycle is called Rapid Eye Movement (REM) sleep. This is the paradoxic, mentally-regenerating stage of sleep. Parts of the brain associated with learning are stimulated, which might explain why infants and children spend a much higher percentage of sleep in REM states. It is thought that REM sleep deprivation impairs memory (NINDS 2005).

> REM sleep begins with signals from an area at the base of the brain called the *pons*. These signals travel to a brain region called the *thalamus*, which relays them to the cerebral cortex – the outer layer of the brain that is responsible for learning, thinking and organizing

information. The pons also sends signals that shut off neurons in the spinal cord, causing temporary paralysis of the limb muscles. (NINDS 2005, 5)

Aside from the eye movements, for which the REM state is named, and associated twitching and movements of the facial muscles, "muscle tone is lost . . . and the capacity to move . . . is eliminated, as are the normal reflexes of wakefulness" (Flanagan 2000, 76). There are often irregular patterns in breathing, blood pressure and heart rate. Emotional centers in the brain often become more active.

Since the early 1950s, REM sleep has been associated with dreaming because subjects who are awakened during this period are easily able to recall dreams (Aserinsky & Kleitman 1953). REM dreams are very active, filled with rich imagery, and possibly responsive to environmental stimuli. They are also often bizarre, illogical and disjointed. In 1962, Foulkes demonstrated that mentation occurs during early stages of NREM sleep as well, but the content is more like waking thinking, "typically dull in imagery, and . . . often a preservative, rut-like theme" (Flanagan 2000, 52).

William Dement, one of Kleitman's students during the 1953 study, is credited with identification of the sleep cycle (Dement and Kleitman 1957), and most early research on REM sleep and sleep disorders (narcolepsy, sleep apnea, etc.). After completing medical studies at the University of Chicago and research at Mount Sinai

Hospital in New York, he moved to Stanford in 1963 to head the first university sleep lab and started the first-ever Sleep Disorders Clinic at Stanford University in 1970. According to Dement, "in the early days of sleep research, there was a de facto prohibition against studying either female subjects or sexual functions during sleep, although the "wet dream," or nocturnal orgasm, was of some interest in its physiological connection to the sleeping brain" (Dement 1992, 134). One of his early observations (mid 1960s), possibly related to an investigation of SRFOs, was that mild REM-sleep deprivation in human subjects resulted in hypersexuality and increased sexual fantasy during waking hours (Dement 1992, 137), suggesting "that REM sleep, and perhaps the concurrent dream-world activities, serve to release sexual tension" (Dement 1992, 122). Dreaming will be discussed in Chapter Five.

A sleeper typically experiences four or five REM periods each night, lasting about ten to forty-five minutes each cycle, with shorter periods at the beginning of the night and longer periods toward morning, for a total of approximately 100 minutes each night (Figure 1). At the end of each sleep cycle, after the REM period is over, there is often a brief period of wakefulness during which the sleeper might look at the clock, adjust the bedcovers, use the bathroom, etc., before rolling over and shifting into the next ninety minute cycle.

Figure 1

Increasing Duration of REM Periods during a Night of Sleep (Dement 1992, 49)

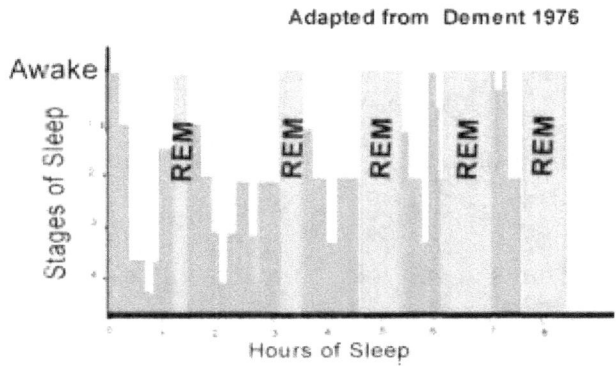

Adapted from Dement 1976

Today, sleep labs use a variety of devices to learn about activity during sleep. In addition to EEGs (electroencephalographs), which provide information about cortical activity, researchers use EOGs (electrocculograms) to record frequency, direction and speed of eye movement; EMGs (electromyograms) to record muscle tone and bodily movement; MEGs (magnetoencephalography) to study sleep oscillations; and fMRI (functional magnetic resonance imaging) and PET (positron emission tomography) to produce images of specific areas of brain activation. PET "shows that limbic activity is high and forebrain activity is low in both REM and NREM sleep relative to wakefulness" (Flanagan 2000, 76).

Sexual Arousal during REM Sleep

The first detailed lab study of male *erections* during sleep took place in 1965 (Fisher, Gross, and Zuch 1965), with seventeen

41

young adult males. "It was found that some form of erection was present in 95 percent of the REM periods (60 percent full and 35 percent partial erections)" (in Van de Castle 1994, 236). A subsequent study by Ismet Karacan, at Baylor College of Medicine, with subjects from age three to seventies, revealed that penile tumescence during sleep decreases with age, but does not disappear in healthy men (Karacan, et. al. 1976). An earlier study by Karacan (1970) "found that subjects with a physical basis for impotence, such as severe diabetes or nerve damage, showed no erections during sleep, while those whose impotence stemmed from psychological causes displayed full erections during sleep" (as summarized by Van de Castle 1994, 236).

In 1983, Fisher et al. published a study of female sexual arousal during sleep using "a thermoconductance method that gives a measure of vaginal blood flow (VBF) . . . [which confirmed] that females manifest cyclic episodes of vascular engorgement during REM periods equivalent to erection in men." These VBF REM increases appeared "to be identical to VBF responses to passive waking erotic stimulation." Therefore, this team concluded that "a very high percentage of VBF REM increases [during sleep] are associated with dreams that contain overt or symbolic sexual content" (Fisher et al. 1983, 97). It probably should be noted that Charles Fisher was a psychoanalyst.

Gary Rogers et al. (1985) conducted a study of female sexual arousal during sleep at the University of Virginia Medical School in 1983. Twenty healthy women participated. A vaginal probe was used to measure vaginal pulse amplitude (VPA) as an indicator of genital arousal. Other physiological measurements (EMG, EEG, EOG), taken from a variety of locations, were also monitored. On the first evening, while in waking states, the VPA showed highly significant changes in response to both erotic visual stimuli and self-directed sexual fantasy. *Interestingly, there was no significant correlation between the VPA measurements and the women's self-rated levels of arousal.* Measurements during sleep were not recorded. During the second night, measurements were recorded during sleep without exposure to the pre-sleep erotic stimuli. "Nineteen out of twenty subjects in this study exhibited VPA increases during REM stage sleep that were similar to those that occurred during waking exposure to erotic stimuli and that were significantly higher than VPA levels during the other stages of sleep" (Rogers et. al. 1985). This group did not assume that arousal during sleep was based on erotic dreams; but instead, emphasized that "self-reported low arousability is not based on lack of physiological response" (Rogers et. al. 1985, 327). This pattern has been rather consistent in research on female sexual arousal.

Both the Karacan and Rogers studies showed that men and women sometimes experience brief periods of physiological sexual arousal during NREM sleep as well as REM sleep. Nonetheless, researchers suspect that most, if not all, SRFOs occur during REM sleep. This is very difficult to confirm. It is extremely rare for male or female subjects to experience nocturnal emissions or orgasms while participating in any kind of laboratory sleep study. In fact, the incidence of sex *content* in dreams is much less in laboratory dream reports than in reports of dreams at home (Hall 1967; Weisz and Foulkes 1970). It is also much more difficult to observe these physiological changes in women than in men.

To date, there has been only one published report of a woman experiencing an SRFO while being monitored in a sleep lab. This occurred during a study on lucid dreaming conducted by Stephen LaBerge. While dreaming will be discussed in a subsequent chapter, for the discussion here it is noted that the fifteen-second orgasm epoch occurred during the REM stage of sleep, with Vaginal EMG (VEMG), VPA, skin conductance level (SCL), and respiration rates at "their highest values and . . . significantly elevated compared to means for other REM epochs. Contrary to expectation, heart rate increased only slightly and non-significantly" (LaBerge, Greenleaf, and Kedzierski 1983).

The data for men are more mixed and inconclusive. Perhaps male sexual responses in sleep are more variable. At least one writer declares that nocturnal emissions occur during NREM sleep (Flanagan 2000, 5), but no supporting research is cited. Other researchers do not specify the sleep stage at which an emission or ejaculation occurred. LaBerge distinguishes between male orgasmic dreams occurring in REM sleep with or without ejaculation, and nocturnal emissions that occur without dreams (LaBerge and Rheingold 1990, 27). A 1983 study of sex dreams in 625 male traumatic paraplegics and quadriplegics documented cases of male sleep orgasm without ejaculation, ejaculation dreams with and without semen evidence, and ejaculation without orgasm (Comarr, Cressy, and Letch 1983).

Interestingly, commentary from both Kinsey's and Masters and Johnson's research distinguishes between male orgasm and ejaculation. Kinsey noted male orgasm without ejaculation among both pre-adolescent boys and adult males, which "physiologically and psychologically . . . may be as satisfactory as those in which ejaculation occurred" (Kinsey et al. 1953, 635). His conclusion was "that sexual arousal and orgasm involve the whole nervous system and, therefore, all parts of the body. Ejaculation is only one of the events that may follow the release of nervous tensions at orgasm" (Kinsey et al. 1953, 635). Masters, Johnson and Kolodny (1982) note this distinction, but view the separation of orgasm and ejaculation as infrequent - the result of disease, illness, youth or advanced age:

> Male orgasm and ejaculation are not one and the same process, although in most men and under most circumstances the two occur simultaneously. Orgasm refers specifically to the sudden rhythmic muscular contractions in the pelvic region and elsewhere in the

body that effectively release accumulated sexual tension and the mental sensations accompanying this experience. Ejaculation refers to the release of semen, which sometimes can occur without the presence of orgasm. Orgasm without ejaculation is common in boys before puberty and can also occur if the prostate is diseased or with the use of some drugs. Ejaculation without orgasm is less common but can occur in certain cases of neurological illness. (Masters, Johnson and Kolodny 1982, 71)

Over the past thirty years, many have debated the possibility of healthy male orgasm without ejaculation in waking states, or even multiple male orgasms. That discussion is beyond the scope of this paper. Regarding the topic of sexual responses in sleep, it will suffice to note that numerous personal reports throughout print and Internet literature suggest that male erotic *dreams* with orgasm *and* ejaculation do sometimes occur during REM periods.

Impact of Drugs and Hormones on SRFOs

Many researchers initially thought that sildenafil citrate (Viagra) would likely be useful in the treatment of female arousal disorders, as it is in male erectile dysfunctions (Berman & Berman 2001, 100-103). Overall, the results have been discouraging, and at this time the pharmaceutical manufacturer has discontinued clinical trials with women. However, several years ago, Rosemary Basson and Lori Brotto (2003), Department of Psychiatry, University of British Columbia, conducted an interesting study to test this drug

46

therapy, which has some relevance to the investigation of SRFOs. A brief summary follows:

Thirty-four post-menopausal women, who had received estrogen replacement therapy for at least six months, were recruited for this study. "Subjects had to meet a diagnosis of acquired genital female sexual arousal disorder, with loss or marked delay and/or diminished intensity of orgasm" (Basson and Brotto 2003, 1015). Rigorous screening and assessment processes, consisting of medical exams, psychological assessment tools, and structured interviews were used to identify a homogeneous subject pool of women who felt sexual desire and responded to non-genital sexual arousal stimulation, but whose genitals had lost sensation or responsiveness to the degree that orgasm was significantly impaired or no longer occurring. Women with neurological disease, dyspareunia, chronic and/or untreated medical or psychiatric illness, hypoactive sexual desire disorder, and various circulatory, and retinal diseases were excluded.

Following the assessment/diagnostic session, the women were divided into two groups, and all participated in a second session that included VPA measurements during and following exposure to an erotic film. The women then completed a self-report questionnaire that assessed mental and physical sexual arousal, and perceptions of autonomic activity and affect. Sessions three and four, in random sequence, double-blinded, included administration of sildenafil citrate or a placebo. After allowing an hour for the drug to work, the women were given a vibrator for clitoral stimulation and instructed to masturbate to orgasm, or discontinue, up to thirty minutes. The women pressed a button at the time of orgasmic release to allow measurement of "latency to orgasm." They then completed more questionnaires.

Overall, the effect of sildenafil on orgasm latency or intensity was not significant. Those with the lowest VPA scores without sildenafil, showed the greatest change in "latency to orgasm," and "older women were more likely to experience orgasm with sildenafil than younger women" (Basson and Brotto 2003, 1019). As with the Rogers study, there was no correlation between women's self-report of mental or physical arousal and the VPA measurements. Interestingly, though, "two women reported experiencing an intense nocturnal orgasm following the session in which they had received sildenafil – such events having self-reportedly ceased more than 10 years previously" (Basson and Brotto 2003, 1018). While this effect is not significant enough to draw conclusions, it suggests that possibly physiological factors, specifically blood circulation in this case, contribute to generation of SRFOs. On the other hand, the study subjects were also exposed to arousal, masturbation and orgasm, all of which, as shown in Chapter Two, have been correlated with SRFOs (Wells 1986; Kinsey 1953).

It is possible that other drugs have an effect on SRFOs, although to date this researcher has located no studies of this effect. A 1998 study by Meston and Heiman showed that "ephedrine significantly (P< .01) increased vaginal pulse amplitude responses to . . . erotic films and had no significant (P>.10) effect on subjective rating of sexual arousal" (Meston and Heiman 1998, 652). Since physiological arousal is associated with SRFOs, it is possible that ephedrine might impact their occurrence.

Other researchers have studied the effects of estrogen and testosterone in treatment of hypogonadal adolescents (Finkelstein et al. 1998). While testosterone was associated with increases in nocturnal emissions in boys, the estrogen did not produce sleep-related orgasms in the girls. This is not surprising since testosterone, rather than estrogen, is the hormone associated with sexual arousal in women as well as men, and arousal is associated with SRFOs.

In addition, to date there have been no published reports suggesting that estrogen replacement in the post-menopausal period increases SRFOs, though it often does improve the quality of sleep and dreaming, by eliminating the "night sweats" which interrupt REM sleep. This is another topic which merits investigation. It is possible that the *active incidence* peak which Kinsey observed was a function of menopause. Perhaps hormone replacement therapy (HRT) extends the active incidence or frequency of SRFOs.

It seems likely that there is a relationship between hormonal activity and SRFOs during pregnancy. Example #6 in Chapter One highlighted this possibility, with the newly pregnant columnist reporting that she experienced SRFOs the three previous nights, prompting her search for more information. (The entire blog for that day, January 24, 2005, is included as Appendix A, since the columnist's comments, and the responses that follow, represent a good cross-section of contemporary public opinion regarding SRFOs and will be referenced as other topics are discussed in this paper. It also includes other pregnancy reports.)

Several other Internet advice columns contain letters from pregnant women inquiring about SRFOs. *Redbook* columnist Janis Graham mentions that "some women do find they're more responsive [to SRFOs] around the time of their period or during pregnancy, when hormones are fluctuating" (Graham 2002), though no references are given. This writer's own recollection is that SRFOs were more common during pregnancy and the postpartum period. Although numerous studies of sleep dreaming (and daydreaming) during pregnancy have been conducted over the past fifty years, it appears that none of them mention SRFOs (Richardson 1996; and Pass, 1996, provide good summaries of this topic). To date, no mention of the relationship between SRFOs and pregnancy has been found in any of the OB/GYN journals.

Similarly, while there are anecdotal reports of SRFO activity being associated with different phases of the monthly menstrual cycle, formal studies, if they exist, have not yet been located by this writer. It is nonetheless widely recognized that "biological conditions unique to women, like the menstrual cycle, pregnancy and menopause, can affect how well a woman sleeps. This is because the changing levels of hormones that a woman experiences throughout the month and over her lifetime, like estrogen and progesterone, have an impact on sleep" (National Sleep Foundation 2004).

A 1966 study (Hartmann 1966) showed a tendency toward longer periods of REM sleep toward the latter part of the menstrual cycle. Other studies have suggested that interruptions in sleep toward the end of the monthly menstrual cycle might account for many symptoms associated with Pre-menstrual Syndrome (PMS) (Pass 1996). Psychiatrist Mary Jane Sherfey, in her influential book *The Nature & Evolution of Female Sexuality* (1966), states that "women are in a mild state of sexual excitement throughout [the 14-day premenstrual] period, although it is rarely recognized as such" (Sherfey 1966, 97). As noted above, arousal is sometimes a precursor of SRFOs. Both Kinsey (1953, 608-10) and Hite (1976, 629) noted that women in their samples reported an increase in sexual desire during this premenstrual period.

Recency of Intercourse or Waking Orgasms Before Sleep

A 1970 study by Karacan, Williams, and Salis has possible relevance for this report on SRFOs. It showed that, for men, recent sexual intercourse resulted in more erections during sleep and shorter periods of time between erections than did abstinence. Overall, recency of intercourse was associated with greater penile arousal during sleep.

This is similar to Kinsey's observation regarding women. He mentions cases "in which the sexual experience of the previous evening supplies the subject matter of the nocturnal dream, leading to a repetition in sleep of the orgasm which had been had before retiring" (Kinsey et al. 1953, 211). He also mentions cases with a high correlation between multiple orgasms while awake and SRFOs. While this suggests a general state of arousal with both psychological and physiological components, it seems possible that multiple orgasms before sleep create a strong physiological predisposition toward SRFOs. Even after stimulation ceases, this physiological propensity lingers. This could be explained by Sherfey's observations regarding labial engorgement, which occurs to a greater degree in women who are more sexually experienced or have borne many children, as a result of increased vascular development (Sherfey 1966, 106-114). "With full venous engorgement and edema [of the labia majora], the plexi and emptied bulbar cavities [which empty during orgasmic contractions] refill immediately" (Sherfey 1966, 105).

> It is in relation to the production of multiple orgasms . . . that the true functioning of the labia majora may be appreciated . . . They act as reservoirs of congested vessels and edema, thereby aiding in the production of multiple orgasms . . . The labia are not emptied during orgasms . . . *Continuous labial congestion and edema constitute a paramount factor in maintaining the sensation of intense perineal and pelvic congestion and of sexual tension* . . . One might say that in the maintenance of continuous sexual tension, the labia majora constitute the "largest plank" in the orgasmic platform. (Sherfey 1966, 107-8)

According to Sherfey, this continuing engorgement of the labia majora allows women to move into a level of arousal where orgasms can continue virtually indefinitely in wave after wave. Sherfey goes on to say, "The more orgasms a woman has, the stronger they become; the more orgasms she has, the more she *can* have. To all intents and purposes, *the human female is sexually insatiable in the presence of the highest degrees of sexual satiation*" (Sherfey 1966, 112).

Masters and Johnson reported that the labia majora (1966, 40), as well as the clitoral shaft and glans (Masters and Johnson 1966, 53) might stay engorged for hours after prolonged excitation, especially in women who have birthed children, when release through orgasm has not been achieved. On the other hand, in private conversation as reported by Sherfey, Masters also hypothesized that frequent high levels of multiple orgasms could lead to a condition of "chronic passive congestion of the pelvis, and work-hypertrophy of the clitoral shaft" (Sherfey 1966, 109-10).

Masters and Johnson reported very few observations about sexual responses in *sleep* for either men or women. However, in their 1982 book with Kolodny, they reported that "testicular aching ("blue balls") in men and pelvic congestion in women may be relieved by orgasms that occur during sleep . . . Although nocturnal emissions ("wet dreams") in young males are well known, females also can experience orgasm during sleep" (Masters, Johnson, and Kolodny 1982, 76). They provide no information or theory about the specific physiological mechanisms which might cause these orgasms to occur. Nonetheless, this statement implies a role for SRFOs in resolving lingering sexual tensions or arousal. Arousal is explored further in Chapter Six.

Physical Intensity of SRFOs

It is not uncommon when discussing this subject to hear women say, "The best orgasm I ever had came as a result of a dream!" SRFOs are frequently experienced as very powerful, often surpassing the physical intensity of waking orgasms. Four of the examples in Chapter One mentioned this intensity. An important key to understanding this is our current knowledge that during REM sleep, voluntary muscle control is lost. As Kinsey noted:

> Sexual responses in sleep may differ, however, from the responses which one makes when awake, in the fact that the learned controls and inhibitions which an individual has acquired in the course of his or her lifetime are less likely to operate in sleep. The content of the dream, the speed of the response, and the abandon of the activity in orgasm may be less obstructed by rational controls . . . One of the most characteristic aspects of nocturnal sex dreams is the speed with which they carry the individual to orgasm, even though he or she may be quite slow in response while awake. An occasional female who finds it difficult to release her inhibitions and reach orgasm while awake may be able to reach it in sleep." (Kinsey et al. 1953, 193)

Lonnie Barbach, a well-known sex therapist, mentions that some of her patients fall into this latter category . . . able to experience orgasm in sleep, but not in wakefulness (in Delaney 1994, 26). Perhaps the speed of SRFOs provides a *surprise* factor, thus enhancing intensity. This could be especially true when there has been no conscious awareness of a preceding dream, as in example #9 in Chapter One. In Kinsey's sample, only 1 percent reported SRFOs without awareness of a dream. The Winokur, Guze, and Pfeiffer study (1959) reported 42 percent in this category; hence, it appears this may happen with some frequency. To go from unconsciousness to a full-blown waking orgasm may be a bit of a shock for some.

Several other factors likely contribute to the experience of intensity. Female orgasm can include not only contractions of the outer third of the vagina, but also of the uterus, and external anal and urethral sphincters (Masters and Johnson 1966, 129-30). The fact that there is nothing in the vagina for the contractions to press against can make them feel much stronger, as though one's entire abdomen is being sucked into a tiny vortex. This can also feel breath taking. While clitoral stimulation during masturbation may produce a similar result, there is obviously some degree of mental preparation while awake, and the unrestrained strength of the contractions in SRFOs often seems greater.

Bladder fullness may also contribute to the intensity of SRFOs. Most women, it is presumed, empty their bladders before sex. After several hours of sleep, the bladder is not empty. Strong contractions, combined with a full bladder, produce a slightly different sensation than typically experienced in coitus. In a very interesting article on *Urethrality in Women,* psychoanalyst Alan Bass points out that in his client practice, "women reported direct sexual stimulation from a filled bladder that men did not experience, and that women also reported urethral masturbatory practices that men did not" (Bass 1994, 491). According to Bass, Freud (*Three Essays on the Theory of Sexuality*) thought that "bladder sensations play a role in nocturnal emissions that is more predominant for women than for men" (Bass 1994, 491). And while bladder fullness might contribute to triggering SRFOs, it definitely plays a role in the sensate experience.

This leads to the idea of female *wet dreams*. Most SRFOs leave little or no fluid evidence. However, there are exceptions. In recent conversations with women, there have been two cases where women reported very large quantities of fluid coming from their genital region following SRFOs. In both cases, this was confusing to the women since the fluid did not feel, taste, or smell like urine. In one case, the woman was so surprised that she was almost convinced that someone had inseminated her. Sex therapists continue to debate the existence and mechanisms of female ejaculation (large volumes of non-urine fluids expelled forcefully from the urethra as a result of sexual orgasm or stimulation ... Ladas, Whipple, and Perry 1982), yet it apparently occurs at least occasionally in SRFOs as well as waking orgasms.

Brain Activity during SRFOs

From the beginning of brain development in the womb, female brains tend to have more connections between the right and left hemispheres. Both dreaming and sexual orgasm have been shown to be primarily right hemisphere functions. The activity of the right hemisphere is responsible for creating, organizing and projecting the dream images, though the left hemisphere is required for memory of the dream (Antrobus and Bertini 1992). "Dreaming, including sexual dreaming, can be conceptualized as a predominantly right-hemisphere function" (Miller 1986). Early research by Cohen, Rosen, and Goldstein (1976) showed that "real, but not feigned, orgasms [are] associated with increased right-hemisphere activity" in both males and females. More recent research by others, including Arnow et al. (2002) for men, and Janszky et al. (2002) for women, has confirmed this.

Some researchers hypothesize "that during REM sleep the connections between the two hemispheres are somehow reduced, allowing the right hemisphere more autonomy of functioning" (Miller 1986). PET "shows that limbic activity is high and forebrain activity is low in both REM and NREM sleep relative to wakefulness" (Flanagan 2000, 76). Consequently awareness and executive control are greatly reduced during sleep.

"The human PET data indicate a preferential activation in REM of the pontine brain stem and of limbic and paralimbic cortical structures involved in mediating emotion and a corresponding deactivation of dorsolateral prefrontal cortical structures involved in the executive and mnemonic aspects of cognition" (Hobson, Stickgold, and Pace-Schott 1998, R1). "The differences between the self-awareness experienced in waking and its diminution in dreaming can be explained by deactivation of the dorsolateral prefrontal cortex during REM sleep" (Muzur, Pace-Schott, and Hobson 2002, 475).

In June 2005, Gert Holstege of the University of Groningen in the Netherlands reported at the European Society of Human Reproduction and Embryology conference in Copenhagen, on his team's recent research using PET technology to study brain response during male and female orgasm (Holstege et al. 2005). As of this writing, the full study has not yet been published. A very brief summary was published in the *Book of Abstracts*, of the International Academy of Sex Research for their July 2005, conference in Ottawa (Holstege 2005a). An earlier PET study of male ejaculation by Holstege's team was published in 2003 (Holstege et al. 2003). This most recent research is the first time that PET brain scans of female orgasm have been obtained.

Due to instrument constraints, the research design required partner-stimulated non-coital, orgasms/ejaculations for both men and women. PET brain maps during female *faked* orgasms and *rest* were also recorded.

> In the female volunteers, in order to be sure that the orgasm was real, blood pressure, ECG, rectal pressure and pelvic floor EMG were also measured. The results show that in both men and women activation was found in the vermis of the cerebellum, and deactivation in the temporal lobe and in women in orbitofrontal and medial prefrontal cortex. Imitating orgasm in women resulted not only in activation of the cerebellum, but also of the genital part of the primary motor and somatosensory cortex, while deactivation, which was so strong in real orgasm, was absent. (Holstege, 2005a)

In other words, it showed that during real orgasm (as opposed to fake), many parts of the brain shut down for both sexes, including the amygdales, parts of the temporal lobes which process fear and anxiety. For women, this deactivation also includes virtually all of the brain parts that register emotion, (conscious or unconscious), the hippocampus, which handles memory (especially emotional memory), and the motor cortex, which controls intentional movement. Movement during real female orgasm is not under conscious control. During fake orgasms, parts of the motor cortex lit up, and the deactivation of the amygdales and other brain structures did not occur. The only part of the female brain to show an increase in activity during real orgasm, was the part of the cerebellum that registers the sensation of being touched or stimulated. This was activated even more strongly in the male subjects.

In response to questions during a recent interview on Australian radio, Holstege made some of the following points: "What I think is the result of our study is how important it is that your level of anxiety or fear has to be in control . . . An interesting thing is that our rational mind is also deactivated during orgasm . . . The conclusion is that this deactivation is really unbelievable . . . In women we saw an enormous deactivation and that was the major thing we found. *De*activation "(Holstege 2005b). This deactivation of the brain strongly supports the idea of orgasm as an altered state of consciousness (Meston et al. 2004), possibly a type of trance or transcendent state, or like a *near-death experience* (NDE) as the French have always contended: *Le petit mort*. Orgasm for women seems to require "letting go" in even more ways than previously suspected.

This study also raises many questions about the operation of the amygdales and temporal lobes, which play important roles in arousal, and will be discussed further in Chapter Six. In these PET studies (Holstege et al. 2003, 2005), male brain response during orgasm was less effectively measurable due to brevity of the male orgasmic response, though preliminary data suggest a slightly different pattern of activity and inactivity.

Deactivation of the pre-frontal cortical structures during REM (Hobson, Stickgold, and Pace-Schott 1998) helps to explain why stimuli that provoke nocturnal orgasms in sleep do not, on their own, usually result in orgasm while one is awake. Since deactivation of these structures is also associated with female orgasm, REM brain conditions are naturally closer to the female orgasmic state. Perhaps this allows the further "brain deactivation," that Holstege sees as a requirement for female orgasm, to occur more easily in sleep.

It is also useful to note that orgasms during sleep are sometimes generated by other brain dysfunctions, especially epilepsy. It has long been recognized that some women experience orgasms related to epileptic seizures while awake. Temporal lobe epilepsy usually produces hyposexuality (Braun et al. 2003). However, *bi-lateral* temporal lobe epilepsy, also known as Kluver-Bucy syndrome, or other cases involving *right temporal lobe* lesions in women sometimes lead to hypersexuality. In a very useful review of brain lesion studies related to sexual drive and behavior, Braun et al. concluded that overall, "hyposexual patients tended to have left hemisphere lesions (primarily of the temporal lobe), hypersexual patients tended to have right hemisphere lesions (primarily of the temporal lobe)" (Braun et al. 2003, 55). In some cases, waking orgasms occur during "partial limbic-temporal seizures" which are also categorized as a type of "ictal alteration" (Ahern 2005, 27). They can also occur during "autonomic seizures," sometimes referred to as "abdominal epilepsy" (Epilepsy Ontario 2005). Orgasms during seizures are more likely when there is also some involvement of the hypothalamus (Ruff 1980). Since seizures can occur during sleep as well as waking states, orgasms have been noted as coinciding with "nocturnal somatosensory seizures" (Calleja, Carpizo, and Berciano 1988). Both waking and nocturnal seizures are usually controlled with anti-epileptic drugs.

A currently popular theory regarding SRFOs (and male emissions) "is that these responses are simply a check to make sure a person's brain, nervous system, and genitals are healthy and in good working order" (Reinisch 1990, 89). This *system maintenance* idea would seem to imply much more regular occurrence with more random precursors than the data throughout this paper suggest. Realistically, a certain percentage of women (approximately 9 percent in Kinsey et al. 1953, 542) never experience an orgasm in their lives, in sleep or wakefulness.

Another popular theory regarding male emissions is that wet dreams are the way the body disposes of old, accumulated semen, to make way for more. Kinsey rejected this theory based on the "fact that females, without testes, prostate glands, or seminal vesicles, still have nocturnal orgasms [thus providing] good evidence that glandular pressures probably have little or nothing to do with nocturnal emissions in the male" (Kinsey et al. 1953, 195). His data for men also showed strong educational, social status, and behavioral correlations relating to nocturnal emissions (Kinsey et al. 1953, 201-2). In addition, there are many men who ejaculate only on rare occasions, for a variety of reasons, without physical harm. Consequently, this theory has not been supported by empirical research.

Waking into Orgasm vs. Staying Asleep - Sexsomnia

As noted above, the Wells study (1986) defined Female Nocturnal Orgasms as waking into orgasm. For purposes of this paper, Sleep-Related Female Orgasms are also being defined as awakening orgasms. Kinsey acknowledged that usually the contractions awaken the experiencer. However, it is possible that these REM-based orgasms might sometimes occur without wakefulness or awareness, leaving only the bed partner as a witness. Kinsey noted:

> The violence of the female's reactions in orgasm is frequently sufficient to awaken the sexual partner with whom she may be sleeping, and from some of these partners we have been able to obtain descriptions of her reactions in the dreams. There can be no question that a female's responses in sleep are typical of those which she makes when she is awake. (Kinsey et al. 1953, 192)

On the other hand, some partner observations might fall into a newly recognized category of sexual behavior now called *sexsomnia*. As noted in the beginning of this chapter, during REM sleep voluntary muscle control is lost, despite the heightened brain acitivity. Paralysis occurs in all of the major voluntary muscle groups. Therefore, dreamers are not able to act out their dreams. For this reason, REM is sometimes called *paradoxical sleep*.

There are other kinds of sleep-related orgasms which occur during the unconsciousness of NREM periods and are more problematic because paralysis of the voluntary muscle groups is not present. In 1996, Canadian doctors Shapiro, Federoff, and Trajanovic (1996) argued that sexual behavior in sleep (when the men or women do NOT wake up) really represents a new kind of parasomnia, like sleepwalking, night terrors, sleep talking, sleep paralysis, etc. These conditions are caused by dysfunctions in the brain wave sequencing of the natural sleep cycle. In 2003, Shapiro, Trajanovic, and Federoff began calling this behavior sexsomnia, although much of the literature also refers to it as *sleep sex* (Rosenfeld and Elhajjar 1998). Beginning in 2005 it will be officially classified as a parasomnia with its own ICSD code (Mangan 2005). Sexsomnia is somewhat similar to sleepwalking and is different than normal SRFOs in that these activities occur during the slow wave phase of NREM sleep; patients are much more physically active; they are totally unaware; and will often initiate sexual behaviors with others. Sexsomniacs have no awareness of the behaviors during the episode or memory of it upon awakening; and it is extremely difficult to awaken them during the event. Often they have a history of other parasomnias including sleepwalking or even sleep-driving. It is thought that more men than women suffer from this condition.

Behaviors initiated by sexsomniacs often go beyond those expressed in waking states. It appears that the most common behavior for women is physically active masturbation accompanied by loud moans and vocalizations. Shapiro, Trajanovic, and Federoff (2003) report that in one "series of patients with sexsomnia, there [was] a high incidence of paraphilic behavioral patterns . . . [They] believe that nonparaphilic sexsomnia is less likely to be seen in a clinical setting. Such nocturnal incidents may be considered as odd but still within present social norms, particularly if the partner is a willing participant" (Shapiro, Trajanovic, and Federoff 2003, 316).

Paraphilic behaviors often include pedophilia with family members or neighbors, exhibitionism, frotteurism, and voyeurism. Sometimes sexsomniacs place themselves at physical risk with resultant bruising or broken bones (Guilleminault et al. 2002). Violent sex and sexual assault during sexsomnia often lead to marital problems and even criminal charges against the sleeping perpetrator. Sexsomnia has been used successfully as a legal defense (Shapiro, Trajanovic, and Federoff 2003, 312; Mangan, 2004) and has been used as a plot line in at least one TV medical show (*House*, 2005). Guilleminault et al. (2002) at Stanford University and Shapiro, Trajanovic, and Federoff (2003) have demonstrated that violent or problematic forms of sexsomnia can be treated with combinations of sleep disorder therapies, including drugs and *continuous positive airway pressure* (CPAP) machines.

Although sexsomnia is a physiological disorder, it often leads to emotional problems for those who suffer from it, even when the behaviors are not extreme. Since the perpetrators are not aware of their sleep behavior, they learn about it from others. A qualitative analysis of 121 reports shows six common themes of reaction: "(1.) fear and a lack of emotional intimacy; (2.) guilt and confusion; (3.) a sense of repulsion and feeling of sexual abandonment; (4.) shame, disappointment, and frustration; (5.) annoyance and suspicion; (6.) embarrassment and a sense of 'self-incrimination'" (Mangan 2004,

287). Obviously, clinicians who deal with sexological issues need to be aware of this disorder.

Sometimes men write to advice columnists, inquiring about the behavior of their sleeping partners. Whether they are experiencing awakening orgasms or sexsomnia, it is interesting that advice columnists from the men's magazines tend to suggest that the SRFOs are serving a compensatory function and can be eliminated if the man fulfills the woman's sexual needs before sleep (Eagan 2004). As has been shown, this is probably not accurate advice.

Use of SRFOs to Retain or Reject Sperm

This perspective on the role of SRFOs comes from the work of evolutionary biologist, Robin Baker, author of *Sperm Wars* (1996). He contends that SRFOs are one of several tools used by women, consciously or unconsciously, to retain or reject sperm from any particular donor (Baker and Bellis 1995), thus ensuring an improved reproductive gene pool. In essence, Baker suggests that women's orgasms, while not necessary for reproduction, have evolved as a tool for selecting the desired donor for conception. The theory is that, through orgasm, women create a "cervical filter" which affects the ease with which sperm can reach the fallopian tubes. This filter consists of cervical mucus, cellular debris, ejected sperm, and other organic material. The strength of this filter varies depending on assorted conditions, including the length of time since last orgasm.

While some degree of filter is developed following coitus with insemination, it declines in efficiency over the next eight days. Through masturbation or SRFOs, or by having an orgasm during foreplay, the strength can be maintained.

In addition, Baker's studies in the lab suggest that the timing of orgasm during coitus has a direct impact on the likelihood of conception (Baker and Bellis, 1995). The cervix dips and opens during orgasm. If a seminal pool is present, the cervix will "suck up" a more significant number of sperm. This kind of "high retention orgasm," defined as one which occurs immediately after partner ejaculation, can override or breakthrough a well-developed cervical block. Female orgasms prior to partner ejaculation "suck up" cervical fluids, increasing the acidity of the cervical environment and strengthening the cervical block. "Thus, a woman can choose, without any conscious awareness or planning, to accept or reject sperm inseminated by a man" (Singh et al. 1998).

Singh et al. (1998) tested this theory with women desirous of becoming pregnant. Their "data support the contention of Baker and Bellis that female orgasm patterning has a significant functional role above and beyond a pleasurable experience. If women indeed utilize orgasm occurrence and its pattern to regulate the amount of sperm retained, the success of such strategy would be greatly enhanced if occurrence of orgasm remained cryptic" (Singh et al. 1998, 29).

CHAPTER 4: BEHAVIORAL FACTORS RELATED TO SRFOs

Although the specific data are somewhat mixed, "there is general agreement that nocturnal orgasms are experienced primarily by women who are sexually experienced; that is, chaste and virginal women are much less likely to experience nocturnal orgasms than non-virgins" (Wells 1986, 422). In Winokur, Guze, and Pfeiffer (1959) only 4 percent experienced a SRFO prior to experiencing coitus, with or without orgasm. On the other hand, it is also important to remember that among Kinsey's respondents, 5 percent experienced their first orgasm, with or without previous coitus, as a result of a sex dream (Kinsey et al. 1953, 193).

Kinsey found that for 10 percent of his respondents, SRFOs began in the same year that other sexual activities (petting, coitus, masturbation, or homosexual contacts) had begun (Kinsey et al. 1953, 210). For 14 percent of his expanded sample there was a positive correlation with lack of social-sexual activity; for 7 percent of his regular sample there was a positive correlation with high levels of sexual activity. He also found a slight positive correlation between occurrence of SRFOs and masturbation, and fantasies during masturbation (Kinsey et al. 1953, 211). Fantasy will be discussed in Chapter Six.

Wells (1986) did not find any correlation between participation in seventeen different sexual activities, or frequency thereof, and SRFOs. This included orgasm, masturbation, and the experience of sexual intercourse. Likewise, Winokur, Guze, and Pfeiffer (1959) found no correlation between SRFOs and frequency of intercourse, frequency of orgasm during intercourse, or sexual satisfaction. Henton's 1976 data, however, suggested that lack of sexual intercourse and social activities among college women were associated with higher occurrence of SRFOs.

Overall, the Wells, Henton, and Kinsey data show some relationship between general sexual arousal or excitement and SRFOs. Since it is sometimes difficult to separate desire and arousal, and arousal has both physiological and psychological components (Palace and Gorzalka 1990), arousal will be discussed as a psychological factor in Chapter Six. It is noted at this point for context.

In summary, the only sexual behaviors that have been shown to have a possible correlation with SRFOs are *lack of sexual activity/opportunity*, *frequent waking sex/orgasm*, and *masturbation*. Therefore, it would be useful to investigate these further.

Low Availability of Social-Sexual Outlets

There are several facets to discussion of this topic, which can be classified into three main categories: biological, behavioral, and psychological. The first issue is biological compensation. As discussed in Chapter Two, this is the notion of a biological process that automatically evokes SRFOs as a way to discharge accumulated sexual energy that is not being discharged through other waking behaviors. Kinsey showed that the incidence and frequency rates of SRFOs for groups without other social-sexual outlets are not nearly sufficient to compensate biologically for the loss of these other outlets. For women who were experiencing SRFOs, at any age, with or without available partners, the frequencies on average, rarely exceeded four or fives times per year. The exceptions to these frequency figures were the women engaged in frequent coital sex and frequent multiple orgasms. Their frequency soared to "at least once a week for at least five consecutive years" (Kinsey et al. 1953, 210).

On average, SRFOs provided the lowest percentage of sexual outlet of any of the sexual outlets studied: "2 per cent of the total outlet of the younger single females in the sample and 4 per cent of the total outlet of the unmarried older females" (Kinsey et al. 1953, 206). The majority of women in Kinsey's sample never in their lives experienced a SRFO, regardless of circumstances. This writer's clinical practice reveals some presumably physically healthy women, usually members of religious orders or older women who have never been in an intimate, sustained relationship, who have never experienced orgasm while asleep or awake. Likewise, there exists a certain percentage of women diagnosed with primary orgasmic disorder who have never achieved orgasm in waking or sleep states (Berman and Berman 2001). These facts stand out as the greatest obstacles to either the *compensatory* or *system maintenance* theories of SRFOs. Therefore, it seems safe to conclude that absence of other available sexual outlets is not enough, on its own, to evoke SRFOs.

Kinsey's data suggest that *previous sexual experience* is an important factor in the generation of SRFOs, although he does not list it separately as a correlated item:

> In the histories of the females who had been previously married, and who in consequence had had their chief source of outlet, marital coitus, more or less suddenly withdrawn, orgasms derived from nocturnal dreams had accounted for a more significant part of the total picture. Among the younger females in the sample who had been previously married, and who were now widowed, separated, or divorced, the dreams had accounted for 4 or 5 per cent of the total number of orgasms. Among the older females who had been previously married, the dreams had accounted for as much as 14 per cent of the total outlet. (Kinsey et al. 1953, 206)

Kinsey assumed that the experience of marriage had increased the *imaginal* ability of these groups. In a later chapter he also hypothesized that "the previously married females may have dreamt of sex more often because of their *desire*, [emphasis mine] conscious or unconscious, for a more active sex life" (Kinsey et al. 1953, 536). While the percentage of total outlet was higher for these *previously married* groups, the active median *frequencies* were not higher than for the *married* groups.

Previous sexual experience, and the combination of *previous sexual experience* with *loss of other sexual outlets* probably are factors in generation of SRFOs, although they did not show up as predictive in the Wells study. Perhaps the college age sample was simply too young and inexperienced. *Previous sexual experience*, on it own, it is not really a biological or behavioral factor. It seems to be more of a psychological factor implying, not only imaginal abilities (fantasy) and possibly desire (as noted by Kinsey), but memory, learning, and enhanced safety with arousal and the orgasmic reflex, as well. It might also be associated with bereavement, since it is not uncommon for women to dream about deceased or divorced spouses in both sexual and non-sexual settings. SRFOs, in these cases, could possibly represent a kind of emotional or psychological compensation.

As noted in Chapter Two, SRFOs provide a higher percentage of sexual outlet for highly educated women at all age levels, especially above age 35 (Kinsey et al. 1953, 563). The role of education will be explored further in Chapter Six, but clearly it too has an impact on imagination, and exposure to ideas. As discussed in the following section, it may also have an impact on sexual skill development and sexual memory development through exposure to a wider range of social-sexual experiences.

Masturbation

Kinsey defined masturbation as "deliberate self-stimulation which effects sexual arousal" (Kinsey et al. 1953, 133). He found that 62 percent percent of the women in his sample had masturbated at some time in their lives, 58 percent to orgasm. Masturbation to orgasm by age twenty included 33 percent of his sample compared with 92 percent at that age in his male sample (Kinsey et al. 1953, 173).

Attitudes about female masturbation have changed significantly since Kinsey's survey. In Shere Hite's 1994 *Hite Report on the Family*, 61 percent of girls surveyed expressed a positive attitude toward masturbation, compared to 29 percent in the 1970s (Hite 1994, 73). *The Janus Report* showed a significant change in attitude among adult women between the Phase One survey (1983-85) and Phase Two (1988-92). "In Phase One, 28 percent of men and 31 percent of women denied masturbation as a normal adult activity; 8 years later these figures had dropped to 12 percent among both men and women. The change in attitude was quite dramatic for women, perhaps as a function of women's learning that masturbation is a societally acceptable activity for themselves as well as for men" (Janus and Janus 1993, 382). Nonetheless, according to the University of Chicago National Health and Social Life Survey (NHSLS) "about half of the men and women who masturbated said they felt guilty" (Michael et al. 1994, 166).

One of the surprising discoveries in both the NHSLS and the *Janus Report* was that masturbation today is often viewed as simply one more expression of sexuality by those who are *already interested in sex and sexual experience*, rather than as a compensatory tool for low sexual outlet. Those with higher rates of other sexual activity, also have higher rates of masturbatory practice and more pos tive attitudes toward it. "It is an activity that stimulates and is stimulated by other sexual behaviors . . . the more sex you have of any kind, the more you may think about sex and the more you may masturbate" (Michael et al. 1994, 165).

Although masturbatory *behaviors* have changed since Kinsey's exploration, the survey results are mixed. In 1976, Hite reported that 82 percent of her self-selecting sample of over 3,000 women masturbated; with 95 percent achieving orgasm "easily and regularly, whenever they wanted" (Hite 1976, 59). In the *Janus Report*, with a representative sample of 1,418 women nationwide, age eighteen or over, 28 percent reported that they never masturbate, and 38 percent masturbated regularly (Janus and Janus 1993, 77). No figures were given for rate of orgasm with masturbation, but 61 percent reported that they always or often orgasm during lovemaking with a partner (Janus and Janus 1993, 86).

The *Janus Report* also found that "the number of women who masturbate increases with education. Those who have never masturbated were 41 percent of the high school group but only 7 percent of the post-graduate group" (Janus and Janus 1993, 295). Although surveys universally indicate that boys and men masturbate more than girls and women, the *Janus Report* found that among adults, "career women approximated the frequency of masturbation for men" (Janus and Janus 1993, 77).

In the 1994 NHSLS survey, with a representative sample of 1,901 women age eighteen to fifty-nine, 58 percent reported that they never masturbated in the past year. This figure seems very high. Of the 42 percent who did masturbate, 61 percent reported that they "always or usually" have an orgasm with masturbation (Lauman et al. 1994, 82). Overall, 71 percent of their sample reported that they "always or usually" orgasm during sex with primary partner (Michael et al. 1994, 128).

For *young* women, the NHSLS (Laumann et al. 1994, 82) reported that 64.4 percent of women ages eighteen to twenty-four, had not masturbated in the previous year, which would mean that 35.6 percent had. This figure is very close to Kinsey's 33 percent "ever masturbated" at age twenty (Kinsey et al. 1953, 173). In the NHSLS survey, masturbatory behavior was also tied very strongly to level of formal education. Only 25 percent of those who had not completed high school had masturbated in the previous year, compared with 60 percent of those with an advanced degree (Laumann et al. 1994, 83). The more educated women also experienced orgasm during masturbation far more frequently, ranging from 45.6 percent for those who had not completed high school, to 87 percent for those with graduate degrees (Laumann et al. 1994, 82). Kinsey's data also revealed the strong impact of education on female masturbation and orgasm (Kinsey et al. 1953, 148-9).

An interesting study by Leitenberg, Detzer, and Srebnik (1993) explored the development of masturbatory behavior in boys and girls during pre-adolescence (before age thirteen), early adolescence (ages thirteen, fourteen, and fifteen), and at college age in 1988. Both male and female groups reported first learning about masturbation through self-exploration (88 percent men, 82 percent women). "Beginning at age 14 more than twice as many male than female respondents said they had masturbated. And of those who did masturbate, the frequency of masturbation was about three times greater for the male than for the female during early adolescence as well as [at college age]" (Leitenberg, Detzer, and Srebnik 1993, 95). Interestingly, the percentages of those who had experienced sexual intercourse by college age (approximately 75 percent) did not display a "gender gap," even though it had existed (35 percent women to 68 percent men, age twenty-one to twenty-five) at the time of Kinsey's survey (Kinsey et al. 1953, 330). Leitenberg, Detzer, and Srebnik concluded that

> Young women in our society simply do not find masturbation as pleasurable or as acceptable as do young men. Yet it has been shown that women can produce an orgasm through masturbation just as reliably as men (Masters and Johnson, 1966). Obviously, despite the similar physical response, masturbation is not as reinforcing for women as it is for men. As pointed out in the Introduction, the usual explanation of this sex difference is that women have been socialized more than men to associate sex with romance and relationships and emotional intimacy . . . What our results may then suggest is that the recent effort to encourage women to take more responsibility for their own sexuality and the explicit suggestion to masturbate more has not altered this socialization process. (Leitenberg, Detzer, and Srebnik 1993, 97)

It appears that *young* women are choosing coitus over masturbation. Although abstinence education may have caused a shift in very recent years, data in the mid-90s *Sex on Campus* survey suggests that college women might actually be surpassing men in percentage of self-reported non-virgins: 81 percent women, 80 percent men (Elliot and Brantley 1997, 5); and frequency of sexual activity: 36 percent of women reporting having sex two or three times a week; 25 percent of men reporting this frequency (Elliot and Brantley 1997, 15). Nonetheless, only 53 percent of the female respondents reported experiencing orgasm "always" or "most of the time" during sex (Elliot and Brantley 1997, 23).

No part of the Leitenberg study defines masturbation as requiring orgasm. Without negating the socialization factors, realistically, as seen in the Kinsey and NHSLS reports cited above, many young women are unable to masturbate to orgasm with regularity, despite the Masters and Johnson results. Likewise, as seen above, many women, especially young women, do not regularly experience orgasm with vagina/penis intercourse. Consequently, while masturbation might be sexually arousing and somewhat pleasurable for young women, the lack of orgasm might make it far less sexually satisfying or self-reinforcing than it is for men.

Since Kinsey's time, surveys on this topic generally show that masturbation becomes more popular with women over time. Kinsey's data showed the active incidences of masturbation were lowest in the younger groups, and highest in the older groups of females. "This increase in the incidence of masturbation among the older females sharply contrasts with the record for the single males where the active incidences reach their peak (88 percent) in the mid-teens, and drop steadily from there into old age" (Kinsey et al. 1953, 143-4).

One reason for this is that orgasm during masturbation *or* vagina/penis intercourse often requires more of a learning process for many women than for men. As theologian and educator Mary Pellauer points out:

> Women cannot take orgasms for granted. Men apparently do so, at least for most of the lifespan.

Female orgasm does not come "naturally." We have to *learn* it. While this may also be true of male orgasm, it is emphatically the case for women. What is learned may be learned askew, idiosyncratically, or may be biased by hidden assumptions. Many layers of interpretation swath experiences of orgasm like veils of shawls. (Pellauer 1993, 150)

Ironically, female orgasm under the age of two has been widely observed and documented (Barbach 1975, 21; Heiman, 1976). Many elements of the cultural socialization process actually train girls/women to suppress the orgasmic reflex, or become fearful of it.

"It is precisely because orgasm is a learned response that therapy programs can successfully treat many sexual dysfunctions. Women who have never had an orgasm, for instance, can learn about their bodies' response to various types of stimulation and increase their ability to have orgasms" (Reinisch 1990, 86). Masturbation provides a wonderful opportunity to learn about orgasm and sexual responsiveness in general; and most women *do* eventually discover their orgasmic abilities without formal therapy or training. Once learned, masturbation is often the most reliable opportunity for orgasm in a woman's life (Hite, 1976).

To the extent that female orgasm is a learned response, as well as reflexive, the statistics cited above show that those with higher education are more likely to find the information and opportunities needed to develop their orgasmic skills during masturbation. Knowledge, comfort and confidence with the orgasmic reflex probably contribute to the frequency and ease of SRFOs, just as they do to orgasms during masturbation and coitus. This would explain why Kinsey found that masturbation was correlated with SRFOs. This relationship is quite different than the current understanding regarding male nocturnal emissions. Young men are sometimes advised to masturbate before sleep as a way to prevent *wet areams* (Reinisch 1990, 91). For some women, masturbating before sleep might actually stimulate SRFOs.

Orgasm Training

Since publication of the Masters and Johnson groundbreaking study of *Human Sexual Response* (1966), and the success of their psychoeducational approach to dealing with *Human Sexual Inadequacy* (1970), a variety of orgasm training programs have been developed, supplemented by a plethora of self-help books. Aside from Masters and Johnson, LoPiccolo and Lobitz (1972), and Lonnie Barbach (1975) made major contributions to this work. Today, both trained professionals and non-professional entrepreneurs conduct these programs. Formats range from individual or couple sessions in a therapeutic context, to work with groups of women, and groups of couples in more public educational or workshop settings. While some programs emphasize specific philosophies, techniques, or even products, most include the following elements and objectives:

a. To provide women with detailed information about female sexual anatomy and encouragement to explore their own bodies.

b. To provide detailed information about the sexual response cycle and typical physiological changes and sensations associated with each stage.

c. To give women permission to think thoughts and have feelings that were previously discouraged, condemned, or even punished.

d. To dispel myths regarding masturbation and orgasm.

e. To encourage women to recognize and value the benefits of masturbation.

f. To create safety and familiarity with personal sensations in response to physical stimulation.

g. To discover personal preferences regarding pleasurable sensations.

h. To develop skill in communicating about personal preferences.

i. To develop familiarity with sensations which trigger the orgasmic reflex.

j. To feel safe "letting go" or surrendering to this reflex.

k. To discover and release possible psychological blocks to "letting go."

l. To develop safety and pleasurable interpretation of the sensations associated with the orgasmic reflex.

m. To feel comfortable experiencing the orgasmic reflex in a variety of settings and conditions; i.e., alone or with a partner.

There are many specific tips, tools and techniques that can be associated with each of these objectives. And, as with many learned behaviors, practice makes perfect. "Sex is actually less instinctive in the human being. Like any other skill, it needs to be learned and practiced" (Barbach 1975, 6). As noted in Chapter Three, the more orgasms a woman has, the more she can have, and the easier and more pleasurable they are.

The ability to experience sexual orgasm provides women with both psychological and physiological benefits. Among these are self-confidence, release of tension, more relaxed lovemaking, self-reliance, increased endorphins, stronger immune system, improved pelvic and abdominal muscle tone, and even healthier skin. As sexologist Diana Wiley says, "An orgasm a day keeps the doctor away!" (Wiley 2005).

One would expect that the popularity of these programs and books over the past thirty years would result in more women experiencing more orgasms more of the time . . . or at least with more reliability during masturbation. While the positive impact of orgasm training with individual participants has been well documented (LoPiccolo and Lobitz 1972), existing survey data make it difficult to discern the cumulative effect in the larger population.

Both the Janus and NHSLS surveys found that masturbatory behaviors were highly conditioned by a variety of social and cultural factors, including education (as discussed above), religion, race and ethnicity. The NHSLS authors recognized that "both women and men had engaged in genital self-stimulation without orgasm. We do not view the absence of orgasm as a behavioral failure; but rather we sense that sexual pleasure is often unrelated to orgasm" (Laumann et al. 1994, 84). Only the Kinsey, Hite, and NHSLS surveys asked about frequency of orgasm with masturbation. In the NHSLS survey, 61.2 percent of women reported "always or usually having an orgasm during masturbation," with those who masturbate most having a higher frequency of orgasm (Laumann et al. 1994, 82-85). "The relation between frequency of masturbation and frequency of orgasm when masturbating is direct. The more often people masturbated, the more likely they are to report experiencing orgasm when masturbating" (Laumann et al. 1994, 84). In 1953, Kinsey reported *accumulated* rates of orgasm during masturbation ranging from 34 percent for women who had never gone beyond grade school, to 63 percent for women with some graduate school education (Kinsey et al. 1953, 148). He did not specify "always or usually." Hite's 1976 self-selecting sample reported a 95 percent rate of "easy and regular" orgasm with masturbation (Hite 1976, 59).

Going back in time, a fascinating study by Katharine Davis (1929) of the sexual practices of 2200 college-educated women showed that, of the women who responded to the questions on masturbation, 62.8 percent of unmarried women over age 18 were able to masturbate to orgasm, with the rate below age 18 being around 13 percent (Davis 1929, 113-115). The nature of orgasm as a learned response, with masturbation providing useful training, was apparent:

> The fact that the percentage of those who never induced the orgasm is so much higher in the group that has stopped the practice [of masturbation] suggests the question whether failure to induce the orgasm has any relation to the discontinuation of the practice. (Davis 1929, 113)

> . . . 32.3 percent of [those] who stopped the practice before inducing the orgasm continued it not longer than six months. (Davis 1929, 119)

> It will be noted that the percentage of those who never induced the orgasm is strikingly larger among those who carried on the practice less than a year – 48.8 percent as compared with 26.2 percent. The numbers, however, are too small to be more than suggestive. (Davis 1929, 121)

Interestingly, the NHSLS "always or usually" rate of orgasm is higher during coitus, 71 percent, than during masturbation 62 percent (Laumann et al. 1994, 115; Michael et al.1994, 128). This 1994 NHSLS rate of orgasm "always or usually during coitus" (71 percent), is above the 1993 *Janus Report* rate of 61 percent (Janus and Janus 1993, 86) and the 1997 *Sex on Campus* rate of 53 percent

(Elliott and Brantley 1997, 23).   Language and data collection differences in the Kinsey, Hite, and Davis studies do not allow comparison.

While conditions of sleep might contribute to ease of orgasm for some women, it would seem also that ease of orgasm in waking states contributes to the incidence and frequency of orgasms in sleep. Orgasm training also raises an interesting question: Is it possible to train oneself to experience sleep-related orgasms intentionally, with reliable regularity? Information in the next chapter suggests that perhaps this is so.

CHAPTER 5: THE ROLE OF DREAMS IN SRFOs

Dreams have been recognized and documented throughout human history. The first recorded dreams are on the clay tablets of the Sumerian Gilgamesh saga, recording data from the seventh century B.C. (Van de Castle 1994, 10-48; Kramer 1969). Dreams have influenced the course of history, and the course of individual lives. Dream tales are scattered throughout the *Bible,* literature, and folk-tales of virtually every culture. Nonetheless, public attitudes toward dreaming have been very mixed. Dreams have been viewed as messages and gifts from God; and also condemned as the work of Satan. They have been valued for healing, problem-solving, inspiration, inner guidance, revelation and self-knowledge; and they have also been viewed as meaningless. They have been encouraged and suppressed. They have been treasured and feared. Since SRFOs and nocturnal emissions occur during sleep, often accompanied by dreams, the history of attitudes toward dreaming has been strongly tied to attitudes toward sex and moral values. The history of these attitudes and moral issues will be covered in Chapter Seven.

Dreaming is a huge topic, about which many volumes have been written. Robert Van de Castle, a pioneering dream researcher and former, long-time director of the Sleep and Dream Lab at the University of Virginia, wrote one of the most comprehensive books on this topic, *Our Dreaming Mind* (1994). It is a well-documented resource including both detailed history and contemporary research for those interested in pursuing this topic. This chapter will focus on contemporary dream research and understandings about the relationships between dreams, sex, and SRFOs.

Theories of Dreaming

An on-going issue in dream research, in general, is the question of whether dream content is primarily compensatory or continuous (reflecting pre-sleep stimuli). To date, studies support both hypotheses, and it is "difficult to design a study in which this issue can be straightforwardly evaluated" (Van de Castle 1994, 256). The problem comes from the impact of imagination itself, which will be discussed further below and in Chapter Six. Human imagination in a waking state produces powerful physiological effects. While this is easily observed in regard to sexual responses, it also impacts other physiological responses. Humans are able to consciously imagine solutions and satisfactions while awake, thus negating the need to compensate in sleep. "So until some way is found to eliminate imaginal activity, conclusions about the effects of presleep deprivation or other conditions to test the compensatory/continuity issue in dreams will remain uncertain" (Van de Castle 1994, 257). Throughout the years, this question has been a significant part of the discussion regarding SRFOs and nocturnal emissions, as well.

There are several different theories regarding the purpose and causation of dreams. Today, these generally fall into four major categories. In this writer's opinion, these are not mutually exclusive. All are probably accurate for some set of circumstances, and individual dream researchers and therapists might incorporate elements of more than one school of thought in their work.

1. Dreaming as a Psychological Process

Surveying contemporary opinion in chronological sequence, the first major category includes those who view dreaming primarily as a psychological process. Sigmund Freud's 1900 volume, *The Interpretation of Dreams*, with eight editions through 1930, popularized this approach. In this view, dreams are seen as a bridge to the subconscious, driven by *wish fulfillment* of suppressed drives (primarily sexual). For Freud, all dreams were symptoms of neurosis. Dream content was viewed as highly symbolic, occurring on both *manifest* and concealed, or *latent,* levels.

> The essence of Freudian dream theory is that dreams are a disguised attempt at wish fulfillment that serve the important function of preserving sleep in the face of episodic pressure from motivational urges like sex and hunger (Freud, 1900). They are disguised by a process called the dream-work, which operates at the behest of . . . censorship. Because the dream-work makes most adult dreams unintelligible, it is necessary to have patients free associate to each aspect of a dream to understand it. (Domhoff 2001)

By the 1930s, Freud acknowledged that dreams might also reflect suppressed fears, anxieties, conflicts, guilt, and trauma. Although he vacillated over the years, he eventually concluded that these too represented examples of disguised wish fulfillment (Van de Castle 1994, 130). While the cause of the dream and the dreaming process might be considered neurotic, subsequent analysis could result in emotional, psychological, and physical healing. Because it occurred as a result of suppressed drives and libidinal energy, it was considered compensatory; allowing "repressed instinctual impulses to be gratified in a hallucinated fashion" (Van de Castle 1994, 128). Freud was a prolific writer who brought dreaming into public awareness and discussion, and emphasized the healing value of dream interpretation and analysis. Nonetheless,

> It could be argued that it is precisely Freud's legacy that has prevented wider acceptance of the full meaning of dreams. Freud forged a strong link between neurotic symptoms and dream formation. No one wants to voluntarily court neurosis. Dreams and sex also became synonymous, and to openly share one's dreams has been considered equivalent of publicly confessing one's private sins and secret sordid desires. (Van de Castle 1994, 138)

Carl Jung, a psychiatrist and life-long dreamer, studied and corresponded intensively with Freud from 1907 to 1913. Jung was also interested in repression and viewed dream content as very symbolic. He held a much broader view of what was being repressed, and preferred to interpret libidinal energy as a more generalized psychic energy, operating with the goal of bringing about a higher order of Self integration. He also viewed dreams as compensatory, though ultimately providing opportunity for parts of the Self that were being repressed to surface into conscious awareness and integration. He referred to many of these parts as archetypes from the collective unconscious. Two soul archetypes, which surface in dreams (often sex dreams), are the *animus*, representing the masculine side of a woman's personality and the *anima,* representing the feminine side of a man's personality. "Jung placed individuation, or the quest for wholeness, as the overarching urge motivating human personality and conceived of dreams as an essential source of guidance toward achieving this wholeness" (Van de Castle 1994, 203).

As a result of Freud's influence, most personality theorists of the twentieth century valued dream awareness and interpretation, even while rejecting many of Freud's specific theories. Consequently, many psychotherapists today include dream interpretation in their repertoire of clinical practices. Elements of Freudian, Jungian, and Gestalt theories are prevalent. "Many contemporary dream therapists have incorporated various facts of Jung's approach without acknowledging, or perhaps without being aware of, their original source" (Van de Castle 1994, 175). In the Gestalt approach, *all* characters and objects in a dream are assumed to represent parts of the dreamer that need to be acknowledged, heard, reclaimed or integrated.

Gayle Delaney's book *Sexual Dreams* (1995) provides other useful insights regarding interpretations of sex dreams. There are many books which focus on more general dream interpretation. One example is *The Complete Dream* Book by Gillian Holloway (2001) employing a database of 18,000 dreams.

2. The Empirical Dream Researchers

The empirical school of dream research emerged in 1953 when scientists, using EEG machines, first associated dreaming with the Rapid Eye Movement (REM) period of the normal ninety-minute sleep cycle (Aserinsky and Kleitman 1953). Armed with new technology, dedicated researchers observed, measured, recorded, and analyzed correspondences between physiology and dream reports. The identification of the sleep cycle, and much of the information in Chapter Three, came from these endeavors.

Many of these early empirical sleep and dream researchers were drawn into this field by their interest in Freudian concepts. For example, Dement felt that his early 1960s observation that REM sleep deprivation in human subjects resulted in hypersexuality and increased sexual fantasy during waking hours (Dement 1992, 134), supported Freud's theory, suggesting "that REM sleep, and perhaps the concurrent dream-world activities, serve to release sexual tension" (Dement 1992, 122). Charles Fisher, who initially studied penile tumescence during REM (Fisher, Gross, and Zuch 1965), and female VBF arousal, (Fisher et al. 1983) was a psychoanalyst.

In 1962, research by Foulkes revealed that some kind of mental activity is always occurring through the night. The NREM mentations tend to be more like waking thinking, often with endless loops of repetitive thought. While NREM ideas *can* be very creative, the REM period experiences are more vivid, distorted, visual, detailed, multi-sensory, or hallucinatory, like a different reality. Nevertheless, since then, there has been a gradual breakdown in the close association between REM states and dreaming. Due to these NREM mentations, some dream and consciousness researchers (Flanagan 2000) now hold the opinion that dreams occur throughout the night. This is one of the current controversies in sleep and dream research (Dement 1992; Domoff 2001). While there are very marked differences between the NREM and REM brain activities, experiential reports from dreamers in some studies show "relatively small REM-NREM discriminability" (Herman, Ellman, and Roffwarg 1978, 90).

Since the 1950s, many researchers have studied dream *content* both in the lab and through dreams written down at home, in response to a variety of manipulated variables. Calvin Hall and Van de Castle developed the first set of statistical norms, *The Content Analysis of Dreams* (1966), which still serves as a reference for those investigating dream content. Gradually, through the 1950s-80s, findings by the empirical researchers began to contradict many of Freud's theories. Comments by G. William Domhoff, a current dream content researcher at the University of California, provide a useful summary of the empirical school perspective.

> As Foulkes (1985) summarized based on a large body of findings, including several of his own studies, dreams are a reasonable simulation of the real world, and they usually concern everyday issues. They are novel constructions, but they usually do not involve highly improbable events. This continuity with waking conceptions and concerns extends to the emotions in dreams, which contradicts one of Freud's key claims about the dream-work...
>
> The similarity between laboratory and home dream reports lends weight to a number of findings revealing that dreams collected outside the laboratory setting usually are far more continuous with waking fantasy and personality test results than might be expected from Freudian claims about the effects of the dream-work. These studies are summarized in two detailed assessments of all the evidence for and against Freudian dream theory by S. Fisher and Greenberg (1977, 1996). In addition, quantitative studies using the rigorous and reliable Hall and Van de Castle (1966) system for the study of dream content have shown regularities relating to age, gender, and culture, and that a person's waking conceptions and concerns can be predicted with a sufficient number of their dream reports (Domhoff, 1996, 2003; Hall, 1947). *Taken together, these findings suggest that dreams reflect or express more than they disguise* [emphasis mine] . . .

In short, a very large body of literature contradicts the claim that dreams are difficult to decipher, and thereby calls the idea of the dream-work or censorship into question. It shows that much dream content is coherent, understandable, and readily related to waking concerns. The main "bizarreness" in dreams is sudden scene changes (Sutton, Rittenhouse, Pace-Schott, Stickgold, & Hobson, 1994), which is not usually thought of as a product of the dream-work. These findings still leave a significant amount of dream content to explain . . .Whatever the exact amount of remaining dream content that is or is not meaningless, however, the important point for now is that the burden of proof is on those who claim hidden meaning to demonstrate their hypothesis with systematic empirical evidence. (Domhoff 2001, 10-11)

In general, the empiricists suggest that dream content is conditioned by the ideas, experiences, memories, and emotions that the dreamer is exposed to in waking states; therefore, it is continuous rather than compensatory. The content is not viewed as particularly symbolic, but is instead viewed as often mundane. These are important concepts when studying SRFOs because they suggest that if one does not think about, or have experience with arousal, sex or orgasm while awake, one probably would *not* have experience with arousal, sex or orgasm while asleep.

3. The Neurophysiologists

This next major classification includes the neurophysiologists and sleep researchers who have tended to view dream production as a brain/biology-driven process. The extreme version of this perspective was epitomized by the Hobson-McCarley "activation-synthesis theory" (1977). In the original version of this theory, the forebrain was simply reacting to signals, "making the best of a bad job in producing even partially coherent dream imagery from the relatively noisy signals sent up to it from the brainstem" (Hobson and McCarley 1977, 1347). In this view, the dream contents were essentially "noise," rather random, incidental, and motivationally neutral as part of a larger maintenance function. Nonetheless, learning, insight, problem-solving and creativity might sometimes result. Hobson and McCarley's significant contribution was in identifying the neural pathways which are activated during REM. But for them, initially, dreaming was a mindless activity totally driven by the pons (brainstem).

Subsequent research by Mark Solms (1997), studying the neural network for dreaming using 361 patients with various kinds of brain lesions, showed that some people with pons lesions still dream, and some do not. The more important area according to his research was the white matter beneath the ventromesial surfaces of the frontal lobe, the frontal limbic white matter. This was an important issue because it allowed a role for conscious and unconscious cognition in dreaming that Hobson's theory did not.

Consequently, Hobson modified his theory, incorporating more of the observations from cognitive/content dream researchers, as well as newer understandings about the role of the forebrain in regulating REM sleep (Hobson, Pace-Schott, and Stickgold, 2000). Among the neurophsysiologists, the role of the forebrain continues to be a hotly debated issue, resulting in increasing distinctions between REM and dreaming (Solms, 2000). Many empirical, cognitive and consciousness researchers are contributing to this discussion (Domhoff 2001; Flanagan 2000; Occhionero 2004).

Another interesting area of exploration for this group is the role of chemical neurotransmitters in possibly highlighting or tagging certain pre-sleep activities or content for further exploration in dreaming (Gottesmann 1999). "Many researchers stress the importance of emotional involvement on the incorporation rate of waking-life experiences into dreams" (Schredl and Hofmann 2003). How are highly focused *cognitive* processes (reading, writing), or the content of such, incorporated into dreams? Much research has focused on the role of acetylcholine and memory. Overall though, this remains an open question (Schredl and Hoffman 2003).

4. The Consciousness Researchers

The fourth major group of theories and opinions comes from the field of consciousness studies, and highlights the opportunities which dreaming provides for consciousness expansion, extending

97

awareness into new dimensions of reality and Self, eventually leading to a higher, larger, more spiritual perspective. Dreams are viewed as doorways to the Divine, offering access to the unified field of consciousness and thus allowing experience beyond the limitations of an embodied personality. From this perspective, precognition, telepathy, revelation and communication with a variety of life expressions become natural.

In recent history, this perspective is often associated with Charles Tart, whose first book, *Altered States of Consciousness* (1969), became a classic from which the field of Transpersonal Psychology emerged. During the 1960s, Tart conducted numerous studies on the use of hypnosis to influence dream activity, which led to other studies suggestive of *out-of-body* experiences. Interestingly though, Freud, Jung and Stekel all strongly "asserted the existence of paranormal dreams" (Van de Castle 1995, 405). In 1920, Wilhelm Stekel (a significant contributor to Freud's understanding of symbology, and a major contributor to the field of sexology as well) actually published a book on telepathic dreaming called *Der Telepathische Traum* (Stekel 1920). Montague Ullman and Stanley Krippner conducted a famous study of telepathic dreaming at Maimonides Hospital in Brooklyn during the 1960s, which they described in their 1973 book *Dream Telepathy* (Ullman, Krippner, and Vaughan 1973).

While this school of thought is listed last, it is actually the oldest by far. Even before the early Greeks went to the temple to dream, humans sought guidance and contact with the Divine through their dreams. The fact that so many dream stories are included in the *Bible* is testimony to this fact. This writer's personal favorite is the story of Joseph, with his *Coat of Many Colors* (Gen.: 37-45), who correctly interpreted the Pharaoh's precognitive dream and saved the kingdom from seven years of famine.

Dream Association with SRFOs

As stated in chapter two, the Kinsey data suggest that, in summary, approximately 70 percent of women have an overtly sexual dream, with or without orgasm, sometime during the course of their lifetime: compared with "nearly 100%" of the males (Kinsey et al. 1953, 215). (This figure for women seems impossibly low to this researcher.) Kinsey also found that SRFOs in his survey were "almost always accompanied by dreams, even among females who are rarely or never given to sexual fantasy while they masturbate or engage in any other type of daytime sexual activity" (Kinsey et al. 1953, 194). He further assumed that the one percent who did not report a dream before orgasm probably were simply unable to recall the dream that had likely occurred. He believed that "the dreams are not only necessary factors in the great majority of cases, but the prime precipitating factors of most nocturnal orgasms," though the influence of physiological factors was recognized as well (Kinsey et al. 1953, 194).

The Winokur, Guze, and Pfeiffer (1959) study found a 42 percent incidence of SRFOs without dream recall. Since this study used clinic patients, there might have been other psychological or pharmacological factors that influenced conscious recall. Realistically, most people do not recall many of their dreams. Nonetheless, since Aristotle's time it has been presumed that dreams likely influence emotional and physiological responses in both sleep and waking states, even when they are not recalled (Van de Castle 1995, 64-5).

It is widely recognized today that dreams recalled prior to SRFOs *or* male nocturnal emissions, often have no overt sexual content (Reinisch 1990, 88-91). Examples #2, #3, and #8 in Chapter One mention this.

Content

It is interesting that very few contemporary dream researchers study the relationship between sexuality and dreaming, despite the physiological sexual arousal that naturally occurs during the REM periods. For example, in reviewing the fourteen year publication history of the APA-sponsored journal *Dreaming* (official publication of the International Association for the Study of Dreams), there is not a single article about sexual dreams or SRFOs. Perhaps this is a reaction to the fervor of the Freudian period where almost all dream content was assumed to be at least symbolically sexual. Or perhaps this relative silence is because some empirical studies suggest that overtly sexual dreams are simply not that common. In a recent email exchange with Robert Van de Castle, he wrote, "Sex dreams are something many people are interested in, but [people in general] aren't willing to share about their personal experiences" (February 28, 2005). In any event, Kinsey is still viewed as the authority regarding frequency and content of sex dreams, and relatively little is known about actual frequency today.

Kinsey presented summary statistics regarding content of the sexual dreams reported by his respondents. Of the 70 percent who reported sexual dreams, with or without orgasm, "between 85% and 90% had had heterosexual dreams;" with 30-39 percent dreaming at least on one occasion of actual coitus; 17-38 percent dreaming of heterosexual petting which did not involve coitus. Eight to 10 percent of the women reported having had homosexual dreams; one percent reported sexual dreams with animals; and 1.5 percent reported sado-masochistic situations. One to three percent reported dreams of pregnancy and childbirth; and about the same percentage reported dreams of rape. Overall, Kinsey's dream content statistics are confusing because individual people have many different kinds of dreams (Kinsey et al. 1953, 213-14).

Kinsey's data suggest that sex dreams "are often a reflection of experience which the individual has actually had;" however, "some 13 percent of the females . . . had had sex dreams which went beyond their actual experience"(Kinsey et al. 1953, 214). The Wells (1986) study found that "dreams were not a significant predictor of nocturnal orgasmic occurrence;" however, "61% reported that their sexual dreams sometimes or always went beyond actual experiences" (Wells 1986, 436).

There have been numerous studies of the dream content of women during pregnancy, and a few studies of dream content during different phases of the menstrual cycle. Overall, dream content during pregnancy can be sorted by trimesters, with self-care issues taking prominence during the first trimester; role and relationship issues dominating the second trimester; and the new child dominating the third trimester (Pass 1996).

> Sleep dreams have been repeatedly cited as reflective of the concerns or problems of expectant mothers. The analysis of content . . . included the expected child, fear of the labor and delivery experience and the ability to adapt to the role of mother. In addition, sleep dreams during pregnancy have been noted to differ from those of nonpregnant women, which seem to support the idea that sleep dreams are related to specific situations and biologic events of daily life. (Pass 1996, 72)

In 1964, Van de Castle (1971) conducted a content analysis of 450 dreams of female nursing students as they related to different phases of the menstrual cycle. While the study is too complex to describe here, some of the findings indicate that images containing blood appear with more frequency during the menstrual period. In addition,

> If nonmenstrual dreams are examined more closely, very different patterns appear for dreams occurring before ovulation and those occurring after ovulation . . .

> The goals during this [preovulatory] cycle phase seem to be receiving attention from males and becoming more closely and romantically involved with them . . .

> The highest level of estrogen secretion occurs during the preovulatory phase . . . *There are more dreams with sex during this phase than any other* [emphasis mine] . . .

> Ovulation occurs at mid-cycle and functions like a railroad switch that moves the dreamer to a new set of tracks. Males, for example, no longer seem so appealing . . .

> The dreamer now begins to gravitate toward other women . . . After ovulation, high levels of progesterone are secreted, and the tendencies toward merger with feminine energy, which began to emerge with ovulation, intensify . . .

> The dreamer has social interaction, aggressive or friendly, with 57 percent of the female dream characters during the postovulative phase, compared to 43 percent during preovulation. The reverse is true concerning male characters. The dreamer interacts socially with only 51 percent of the male dream characters after ovulation,

compared to 82 percent during the preovulative and 85 percent during the premenstrual phases . . .

In dreams during the premenstrual phase, interpersonal relationships are very ambivalent, unsatisfying, and often involve triangular relationships with feeling of jealousy. A high density of male characters appear, but they are frequently dating other women and leaving the dreamer behind . . .

Sexual encounters generally had an unfortunate outcome in premenstrual dreams...

It is critical in any study of women's dreams to take the menstrual cycle into account, because dream scores can shift so dramatically form one phase to another. (Van de Castle 1994, 382-8)

It is interesting to note that while sex dreams occur more frequently during the preovulatory phase, sexual arousal and SRFOs might be more common during the postovulatory, premenstrual phase as noted in Chapter 3. This would suggest that sex dreams alone are not strongly predictive of SRFOs, as found in the Wells (1986) study cited above.

The 1966 Hall and Van de Castle study, *The Content Analysis of Dreams,* analyzed the dream content of 1,000 dreams of college students (five dreams from each of 100 male and 100 female dreamers). The purpose was to identify quantitative norms for a variety of subject scales and categories. In general, the women reported more human characters in dreams than did men, and more personal emotions.

Interestingly, the number of reported sex dreams for women (in which they participated in sex) was very low: slightly over 3 percent for that age group during that particular dream series, and definitely less than the12 percent reported for males. (Women reported slightly higher numbers than men of dream incidents where they observed others having sex.) One result of this study was the "generally accepted notion about the differences between the dreams of men and women . . . that men's dreams have more manifest (frank) sexual content or imagery than do women's dreams" (Delaney 1994, 4). Later studies by Kremsdorf et al. (1978) at the University of Arizona, and Robbins, Tank, and Houshi (1985) at George Washington University, refuted this, and showed no difference in the intensity or degree of sexual content of male and female dreams. This change seems to correspond with the significant increase noted in Chapter Two in incidence of SRFOs among college women during the time period of the cultural *sexual revolution.*

In discussing content, dream therapist Gayle Delaney, author of *Sexual Dreams* (1994, reprinted as *Sensual Dreaming*) points out that:

> Our sexual dreams are generally quite different from our sexual fantasies in several ways. Our sexual fantasies are usually erotically exciting, they unfold in a predictable manner, and they follow a fairly uncomplicated story

line. Our sexual dreams, on the other hand, are sometimes not at all erotically exciting; there are usually all sorts of surprises, interruptions, and twists in the plots; and the story lines can be very complex indeed. Most of us call up sexual fantasies to turn us on, whereas our dreams come unbidden and sometimes shock the daylights out of us . . . Our dreams tell a story in pictures about how we feel about our sexuality and about our sexual relationships. They go much further than fantasies; they show us when we are in trouble, how we got there, and they give us the understanding to work our way out of our difficulties. (Delaney 1994, 7-8)

While Kinsey felt that his data did not add to any discussion of dream symbolism, he noted that "not a few individuals derive considerable pleasure from vicariously participating through these dreams, in activities which, for one reason or another, are unattainable in actual life" (Kinsey et al. 1953, 214). He also mentioned that, compared to men, women worry less about their sex dreams, and accept the experiences as pleasurable.

It is not the purpose of this paper to analyze dream content or symbolism. It will suffice to say that anecdotal evidence suggests that women's sex dreams today contain the same kinds of experiences that Kinsey reported: heterosexual, homosexual, and animal contacts; coitus, petting, and self-pleasuring. The pleasurable "dream characters" often include former lovers/spouses, famous people, characters from fiction (TV, movies, books), unknown or mysterious characters, and mildly coercive or forceful men/partners

(Delaney 1994, 13-31). Here is a summary report from a recent conversation with a middle-aged woman:

> The first sexual dream I recall was at age 4. I guess I was into anal sex and "golden showers" at that stage, or perhaps I just hadn't yet discovered my clitoris and vagina. But I definitely remember the sexual feelings. Throughout childhood many of my sexual dreams involved TV characters, especially cowboys, and the Lone Ranger showed up well into my college years. "Who was that masked man?" Over the past twenty years or so, Richard Gere has surprised me with pleasant dream visits numerous times. "Shall we dance?"

Unpleasant sex dreams often include sex with family members or unattractive people, embarrassing situations, being interrupted or "caught," or threats of violence. While rape fantasies might be experienced as pleasurable, rape dreams usually are not. Unpleasant sex dreams do not usually result in orgasm (Delaney 1994). *On the other hand, as noted above, orgasm sometimes comes without any awareness of a dream, or as the result of a dream that does not appear to have any sexual content whatsoever.*

Our culture today allows women much more freedom to acknowledge and talk about sex dreams. Recently a heterosexual female TV sit-com character mentioned that she had had one of her "lesbian orgy dreams" the previous night (*Committed* 2005). The context of the comment indicated that this was a normal, pleasurable, even exhilarating, experience.

Dream Incubation

There are a variety of techniques in use for gaining more conscious control of one's dream experiences. Perhaps the most popular is "dream incubation." This has been practiced in almost every civilization and culture, both East and West, usually as part of healing or spiritual rituals. "Mesopotamians and Egyptians practiced dream incubation, but under the Greeks, the practice became a highly developed art " (Van de Castle 1994, 62).

Dream incubation is a tool for accessing inner guidance. As practiced today, with numerous variations, the dreamer essentially asks a question, states a problem, or makes some other kind of request before sleep. The answer, solution, information, or requested experience is revealed in a dream. A fairly standard formula for dream incubation is published on Gillian Holloway's web site: www.lifetreks.com/lifetreks2/incubation.asp, and is included as Appendix A. Most practitioners obtain satisfactory results with dream incubation rather quickly. Many modern day scientists, inventors, artists, writers, etc., credit dreams and intentional dream incubation for their success (DeAngelis 2003).

It is actually possible to use the dream incubation process to induce SRFOs, both directly and indirectly. Example #1 in Chapter One could be considered the result of dream incubation. The question in this writer's mind was whether to use the designation "female nocturnal orgasm" for this paper despite its inaccuracy, or switch to a different designation. The dream guidance was quite clear, and included an unexpected SRFO.

Today, Internet web pages include a variety of suggested, yet uninvestigated, techniques for "the popular cultivation of orgasmic dreams" (Steward 2002, 26). Following up on Tart's early research, some Internet writers/entrepreneurs suggest seeking SRFOs directly through hypnosis or self-hypnosis (Friesen 2003). On the other hand, some people are highly suggestible most of the time. During a recent business trip, this writer casually discussed this dissertation topic over lunch with a workshop participant (mid 40s, married, mother, graduate school education). The next morning she said, "Wow! I think you need to talk with me some more! Last night I had one of those orgasms in my sleep. It was amazing. And I don't really know how to say this . . . it was so intense!" Wells (1986) raised the issue of *suggestibility*, as discussed in Chapter Two. Perhaps this is one reason why women are not taught about SRFOs.

Lucidity and Volition

Lucid dreaming has been described in literature at least since St. Augustine in 415 A.D., and has been part of the spiritual training in the Tibetan Buddhist and Islamic traditions, as well as the spiritual training of many more primitive cultures, including Native Americans. In recent decades it has become a popular tool in Western spiritual and consciousness explorations. The term is attributed to Dutch psychiatrist Frederik Van Eeden who presented a paper in 1913 at the Society for Psychical Research. He used this term to describe dreams in which he was aware that he was dreaming, had full recollection of his day life, and "could act voluntarily" within the dream (Van de Castle 1994, 440-1).

Normally, this latter quality of *volition* is an essential element in the definition of lucid dreaming. However, some dream therapists, like Delaney (1994) and Holloway (2001), use this term to mean simply that "you are aware of the fact that you are dreaming while you are asleep having the dream" (Delaney 1994, 26). This is an important distinction, and for purposes of this discussion, the element of volition will be assumed.

Aside from volition, "lucid dreams are often distinguished by the greatly enhanced sensory awareness that appears in them" (Van de Castle 1994, 443). At times, the sensory awareness is so great that lucid dreamers throughout history have often designated this state as another reality. Stephen LaBerge presents a highly useful discussion of this topic in Chapter Nine of his groundbreaking 1985 book, *Lucid Dreaming*. A result of this condition is that, "Women sometimes have quite vivid sexual dreams in connection with nocturnal orgasms, so much so that on occasion the dreamer may believe she has actually had sex" (Adams 1981).

Lucid dreaming was first demonstrated in a British sleep lab (Hull University) in 1975, and in Stanford University Sleep Lab by

Stephen LaBerge in 1980 (under guidance from Dement). It took awhile for either study to be accepted for publishing. In 1981, LaBerge presented four papers on lucid dreaming at the Association for the Psychophysiological Study of Sleep meeting in Massachusetts. Since then, LaBerge has conducted much research through the Lucidity Institute, and published extensively. Today there are many books about lucid dreaming, by many authors. Typically these books also teach techniques for cultivating lucid dreaming skills (Van de Castle 1994, 444-448).

LaBerge's studies require that subjects in a sleep lab, attached to various physiological monitoring devices, provide a particular ocular signal (side to side eye movements) every ten seconds to indicate when they are aware that they are dreaming. Obviously this requires awareness and volition. The most exciting and satisfying part of lucid dreaming comes from the dreamer's ability to influence the course of the dream events. *Influence* does not mean total control; however, the ability to participate in an interactive manner leads to interesting experiences and awareness.

Delaney comments that many of her clients and students report that "a number of their orgasmic dreams are lucid ones" (Delaney 1994, 26). Patricia Garfield, author of *Creative Dreaming* (1974) and *Pathway to Ecstasy* (1979) writes that:

> When you become lucid you can do anything in your dream. You can fly anywhere you wish, experience love-making with the partner of your choice, converse with friends long dead or people unknown to you; you can see

any place in the world you choose, experience all levels of
positive emotions, receive answers to questions that
plague you, observe creative products, and in general,
use the full resource of the material stored in your mind.
You can learn to become conscious during your dreams.
(Garfield 1974, 143)

Even without training, many people experience lucid
dreaming. A study by Deborah Armstrong-Hickey reported that lucid
dreaming is apparently quite common in childhood and decreases
with age, especially during the period of age 10 to 12 (Armstrong-
Hickey 1991, 250-54). Interestingly, brain wave activity also shifts
dramatically during this developmental time, with the beta
frequencies becoming the dominant waking signals. And obviously,
this period also corresponds to sexual puberty.

In 1989, Jayne Gackenbach estimated, on the basis of various
studies she had conducted, that:

About 58% of the population have experienced a lucid
dream at least once in their lifetime, while about 21%
report it with some frequency (one or more per month).
Additionally, 13% of dreams recalled on the morning
after and recorded in dream diaries are likely to be lucid.
(Gackenbach and Bosveld 1989, 91-92)

Given the interest in tools for developing lucid dreaming, these
figures might be higher today. Increases in lucid dreaming have been
reported with hypnosis (Dane and Van de Castle 1991), self-hypnosis,
autosuggestion, brain-wave training, and meditation techniques,
especially among women (Gackenbach 1990). As Stewart points out,

112

"The techniques for achieving lucidity are neither mysterious nor excessively demanding. Many report their first lucid dream experiences after merely learning about the idea (Green & McCreery, 1994)" (Stewart 2002).

LaBerge's 1983 study, reported in Chapter Three, included female orgasm during sleep in a sleep lab, and occurred during a lucid dream experiment. Prior to going to sleep, the subject had been instructed to initiate sexual activity in her dream after becoming lucid. During the study, she signaled with eye movements when she became lucid. She then gave the agreed-upon signal when she initiated sexual activity. This resulted in a fifteen-second orgasm epoch during the REM period of sleep (LaBerge, Greenleaf, and Kedzierski 1983).

Lucid dreaming and consciousness training in general have a significant impact on our discussion of SRFOs. Patricia Garfield, one of the most adventurous writers regarding the lucid dream state says:

> My present hypothesis is this: *Orgasm is a natural part of lucid dreaming.* My own experience convinces me that conscious dreaming *is* orgasmic. Too many of my students have reported similar ecstatic experiences during lucid dreams to attribute the phenomena to my individual peculiarity. There is a kind of mystic experience involved . . . I believe it quite possible that in lucid dreaming we are stimulating an area of the brain, or a chain of responses, that is associated with ecstatic states of all sorts. Sensations of flying, sexual heights,

acute pleasurable awareness, and a sense of oneness are all natural outcomes of a prolonged lucid dream.

In my early experiences of conscious dreaming I woke immediately prior to, during, or after orgasm. Now I've learned to stay within that special space moments longer and explore it further. (Garfield 1979, 44-45)

Recent research on neural pathways associated with both dreaming and female orgasm would seem to support Garfield's hypothesis (see Chapter Three). Overall, she reports that about two-thirds of her lucid dreams have sexual content, and about half of these culminate in orgasms of profound intensity. Interestingly, LaBerge states that women report more orgasms from dreams than do men (LaBerge and Rheingold 1990, 26). However, he distinguishes between male orgasms and *wet dreams* (which often are not accompanied by dreams). According to LaBerge,

There are both psychological and physiological reasons why the lucid dreaming state tends to be a hotbed of sexual activity. In terms of physiology, our research at Stanford has established that lucid dreaming occurs during a highly activated phase of REM sleep, associated, as a result, with increased vaginal blood flow or penile erections. These physiological factors coupled with the fact that lucid dreamers are freed from all social restraint ought to make lucid dream sex a frequent experience. These findings imply that lucid dreaming could become a new tool for sex therapists, and new hope for those who suffer from some forms of psychosexual dysfunction . . . Like many new ideas . . . this is untested and ripe for research. (LaBerge and Rheingold 1990, 171)

CHAPTER 6: OTHER PSYCHOLOGICAL AND BEHAVIORAL FACTORS RELATED TO SRFOs

This chapter will highlight more of the data regarding factors that have been identified as correlated with, or predictive of, SRFOs.

Overall, these factors include: *masturbation* (Kinsey et al. 1953) which was discussed in Chapter Four, *fantasy during masturbation* (Kinsey et al. 1953), *orgasm through fantasy alone* (Wells 1986), *satisfaction with one's sex life* (Wells 1986), *high levels of erotic responsiveness (arousal)* (Kinsey et al. 1953; Henton 1976; and Wells 1986), and *anxiety* (Wells 1986; Henton 1976; and Winokur, Guze and Pfeiffer 1959). *Low levels of social-sexual outlet* (Kinsey et al. 1953 and Henton 1976), *desire* (Kinsey et al. 1953), and *previous sexual experience* (implied in Kinsey et al. 1953) were discussed in Chapter Four. In addition, *sexual liberalism, waking sexually excited from sleep, being familiar with the phenomenon of nocturnal orgasms, and/or having a positive attitude toward nocturnal orgasms*, were identified by Wells (1986). In discussion, Wells also wondered about the role of *suggestion*, mentioned in Chapter Five. In Chapter Two, it was suggested that *formal education* might also be a relevant factor.

Education

When discussing men, Kinsey noted that "the males who go furthest in their educational career appear to have better developed imaginative capacities, and this seems to have an effect upon the development of their psychosexual responses," thus perhaps accounting for their higher frequencies of sex dreams and nocturnal emissions (Kinsey et al. 1953, 201-2). Kinsey did not observe this relationship for women, although, his data for women, especially women with graduate school education, seemed to support a connection (See Chapter Two).

Chapter Two included additional statistics and discussion suggesting that education might be a factor in the incidence of SRFOs. The Henton (1976) and Wells (1986) surveys included only college women in their samples. Both studies showed incidences of SRFOs well above Kinsey's data for that age. They also suggested that the incidence of SRFOs in the college-age population was increasing rapidly during the 1970-80s period, strongly influenced by cultural factors.

The Wells survey showed a positive correlation between SRFOs and *being familiar with the phenomenon of nocturnal orgasms, and/or having a positive attitude toward nocturnal orgasms.* Despite the higher levels of sexual activity among more educated women, there is no data that specifically suggests that they are more likely to have knowledge of SRFOs. None of the major surveys have addressed this topic; and in the Wells study (1986), 35 percent of the respondents had never heard of SRFOs. This writer's informal survey places this figure in excess of 25 percent today. While it is possible that this topic might be covered in coursework along the way, it is likely that women learn about SRFOs from experience and, based on experience, develop a positive attitude toward them.

Nonetheless, it appears that formal education has a tremendous impact overall on women's sexual experience, expression and attitudes. For example, Chapter Four presented data showing that masturbation rates and ability to masturbate to orgasm were more frequent among educated women. The *Janus Report* found that "women with the highest education report having the greatest number of sex partners – twice as many as any other group of women – and the most sexual experience before marriage" (Janus and Janus 1993, 295). The *Sex on Campus* survey showed college women leading the men in frequency of going "all the way" (Elliot and Brantley 1997, 15).

By comparison, according to the *Janus Report*,

> The women in the high school group seemed, in our data, to be locked in a tiresome existence. One sees dramatic evidence . . . that the high school educated females consistently showed a greater lack of sexual development, of experience, and of sexual growth, compared with either the men in the high school group or the other women. Our image of the high school

educated woman is that, compared to the other women, she feels the least sensual, is the least sexually active, has had the least premarital sexual experience, is the most passive, and has the least interest in professional attainment. She is also against (and fears) divorce, and she shows the least awareness of the sexual double standard." (Janus and Janus 1993, 321)

While the impact of education on the incidence or frequency of SRFOs has not been adequately studied, it would seem that there is a logical connection. Education provides exposure to many diverse ideas, as well as stimulation and development of the creative and discriminative mental faculties. The milieu of campus life during an important psychosexual developmental stage provides abundant opportunity for experimentation and exploration. Educational differences show up in sexual behavior throughout the lifespan, with more highly educated women continuing sexual activity into an older age (Janus and Janus 1993, 321). Kinsey's data showed this to be true of SRFOs also with the highly educated ("17+" years) group being the only *single* women educational level category to continue SRFOs past age forty (Kinsey et al. 1953, 218), and SRFOs representing a higher percentage of sexual outlet for highly educated women at all age levels, especially above age 35 (Kinsey et al. 1953, 563). "Those with more education – most dramatically, the women in the postgraduate group – showed a greater ability to make choices and to enjoy a more varied diet of sexual experience . . . they report much greater gratification in their sexuality" (Janus and Janus 1993, 321).

Higher education has a life-long impact on sexual attitudes, behavior, waking experience, imagination, motivation, and arousal. This might be sufficient to trigger SRFOs at a rate in excess of that experienced by less educated women. This is an untested hypothesis. The specific nature of the connection is unclear. Do well-educated women think about sex more than the less educated? If one is thinking about sex when awake, it is likely that sex will also appear in sleep-time mentations and images according to empirical research about dreaming. Are well-educated women more sexually aroused? Or does higher education have its impact by removing cultural myths and fears about experiencing sexuality?

Personality Factors

Underlying this behavioral data is the more basic issue of personality. Who are the women attracted to higher education to begin with? What qualities do they bring to the educational experience? What qualities to they seek to develop further? While the experience of formal education might contribute to SRFOs, it is also possible that the true predictors are *personality characteristics* that have not yet been studied at all in relationship to SRFOs. Chief among these would be self-confidence, competence, self-reliance, self-expression, creativity, assertiveness, adventurousness, and general tendencies toward self-actualizing, inner-directed motivation and generally good mental health.

Numerous studies since the 1930s have shown that women who rate highly on these personality factors are more orgasmic. Seymour Fisher, in his book *Sexual Images of the Self* (1989, 49-50) presents a good summary of these studies, and concludes by declaring "that active women are more effective in reaching orgasm than are passive women" (Fisher 1989, 50). Abraham Maslow, a humanistic personality theorist who studied happy, healthy, "self-actualizing" women in the 1930s-40s, was of the opinion that orgasmic sexual dreams are "characteristic of women who are self-assured, poised, independent and generally capable. Women with low self-esteem (who are more inhibited) usually have romantic, symbolic, anxious, or distorted sexual dreams, he found, compared to open dreams of the sexual act by women with high self-esteem" (Maslow 1942, summarized in Garfield 1979, 126).

Given that incidence of SRFOs continues to increase with age, it is also possible that these experiences are products of a psychological maturation process which might lead to eventual development of the personality factors mentioned above, with or without formal education.

It also seems possible that SRFOs might be a basic indicator of intelligence. This notion comes from the fact that in Kinsey's sample, the women who eventually sought graduate school education often reported experiencing SRFOs at younger ages than less educated groups (Kinsey et al. 1953, 218). Higher education would not yet have taken place, and consequently the effects thereof would not yet have had an impact. Likewise, higher intelligence is often associated with the personality factors mentioned above. Fisher's discussion actually begins with mention of the famous Terman longitudinal study of 1300 high IQ children, which concluded that high IQ test scores were correlated with greater physical and mental health (Terman and Oden 1959). This is an interesting and totally untested hypothesis.

Attitudes

In 1986 Wells commented,

> That liberal sexual attitudes and positive attitudes toward nocturnal orgasms are strongly associated with their occurrence appears to indicate that the removal of prohibitive sexual attitudes may increase one's awareness of and/or reporting of nocturnal orgasm experience. Nonetheless, one must wonder which comes first, the nocturnal orgasm or the liberal sexual attitudes. Is the experience of nocturnal orgasm conducive to the development of liberal sexual attitudes or does possessing prosexual attitudes facilitate having this erotic sleep activity? (Wells 1986, 434)

Attitudes are closely related to both personality factors and behavior. Data from the NHSLS and the *Janus Report* show dramatically more liberal sexual attitudes among educated women, and a tendency toward more liberal sexual attitudes in many categories (especially toward variety of sexual behaviors), for men and women overall since the time of Kinsey's survey. In addition,

> [The NHSLS] found that there is a strong, robust link between attitudes and sexual behavior, and that it suggests why so many social issues related to sex are so contentious. Not only do people's underlying attitudes about questions of sexual morality predict what sort of sex they have in the privacy of their bedrooms, but they even predict how often people *think* about sex. (Michael et al. 1994, 321)

And if thinking about sex when awake, leads to thinking about sex in dreams/sleep, as suggested by the empirical dream studies, then indeed *prosexual attitudes* would be a useful predictor of SRFOs. If "prosexual attitudes facilitate having this erotic sleep activity," one would have to assume that the incidence and frequency of SRFOs would have increased greatly since Kinsey's time. However, given that a substantial percentage of women do not even know about SRFOs, they obviously do not have any attitude toward them, as discussed above.

Wells states that *"satisfaction with one's sex life* [emphasis mine] was a significant predictor of ever having experienced nocturnal orgasm and having experienced nocturnal orgasm within the past year" (Wells 1986, 432). Nonetheless, the actual data regarding this factor is rather mixed; and different assessment instruments related to this factor produced different results.

Winokur, Guze and Pfeiffer (1959) found no correlation with sexual satisfaction. This might be one of the primarily psychological factors which Kinsey thought could act in different ways at different times (Kinsey et al. 1953, 211), although he did not specifically report on sexual satisfaction relative to SRFOs. Perhaps *both* satisfaction and dissatisfaction are predictive of SRFOs. One might assume that Kinsey's 7 percent high waking orgasm/high SRFO group felt satisfaction with their sex life. One might also assume that his group of prison inmates and widows felt overall dissatisfaction. Therefore, familiarity with current statistics regarding sexual satisfaction is probably useful, despite the direction of the correlation with SRFOs.

In earlier surveys women reported the following levels of being *very* satisfied with their sex lives: *Janus Report*, 1993: 44 percent at "biological maximum" (Janus and Janus 1993, 93); NHSLS, 1994: 40 percent (Michael et al. 1994, 124); *Sex on Campus* (young women), 1997: 45 percent (Elliot and Brantley 1997, 12).

Interestingly, of the surveys mentioned above, only the *Sex on Campus* survey provides clear data on dissatisfaction with sex life, with 15 percent of the young women reporting to be "not very satisfied" (Elliot and Brantley 1997, 12). A "National Survey of Women in Heterosexual Relationships" conducted by Bancroft, Loftus, and Long of the Kinsey Institute (2003), showed 24.4 percent of women reporting "marked distress about their sexual relationship and/or their own sexuality" (Bancroft, Loftus and Long 2003, 193).

This was a telephone poll using a structured interview based on a national probability sample of 987 women. "The best predictors of sexual distress were markers of general emotional well-being and emotional relationship with the partner during sexual activity" (Bancroft, Loftus and Long 2003, 193).

Fantasy and Imagination

Kinsey noted that *fantasy during masturbation* was positively correlated with incidence of SRFOs. Overall, he defined fantasy as becoming erotically "aroused by thinking of sexual relations - by thinking of the sexual relations that [one] had previously had, or by thinking of the sexual relations that [one] might anticipate having or would like to have" (Kinsey et al. 1953, 665). In his study, 62 percent of the women reported masturbating (Kinsey et al. 1953, 173), and 64 percent of this group reported that fantasy accompanied masturbation (Kinsey et al. 1953, 164). Fantasies were more common among older women, and overall, women in his sample rarely fantasized activities that were beyond or outside of their experience (Kinsey et al. 1953, 164). While masturbation rates for women were related to education, Kinsey did *not* find a relationship between female sexual fantasy and education. Kinsey concluded that fantasy was less important for female sexual response than it appeared to be for men, who reported 89 percent fantasy during masturbation (Kinsey et al. 1953, 667). He went on to report, "We have nearly no cases of females utilizing erotic books or pictures as sources of stimulation" (Kinsey et al. 1953, 668).

Understanding of the role of sexual fantasy has changed significantly in the years since Kinsey's study. Both Freud (1905) and Reich (1942) considered sexual fantasies to be signs of neurosis or sexual maladjustment. Historically, clinicians valued sexual fantasies only as tools for assessing pathology; and fantasy during sexual intercourse was considered a form of masturbation. This started to change during the 1960s and 1970s. Increasingly clinicians began to recognize the very important role that the mind plays in sexual desire and arousal. Heiman, LoPiccolo and LoPiccolo, authors of *Becoming Orgasmic,* concluded that fantasy can not only enhance arousal and help women feel sexier, but it can also limit distractions that might interfere with sexual enjoyment. It is a tool that empowers women to take more responsibility for *turning themselves on* rather than being dependent on a partner or circumstances (Heiman, LoPiccolo, and LoPiccolo 1976, 79-84, 152-155). "Sexual pleasure means involving your body *and* your mind. Fantasy is one way to do this" (Heiman, LoPiccolo, and LoPiccolo 1976, 79).

David Schulz, in his 1984 book *Human Sexuality*, points out:

Human sexuality is to an unknown extent a creation of the human mind . . . our pluralist society contains a complex set of beliefs, attitudes, images and emotions that help define what human sexuality is for a particular person. This complex gestalt is said to be held in the mind . . .

There is nothing that will automatically arouse us . . . human sexual arousal is not a reflex response for either men or women. The male is frequently aware of the effect of mental images in stimulating an erection, and more women are reporting comparable effects upon vaginal lubrication. Nevertheless, not all persons are aware of these images, and not all report sexual fantasies even though they are fully aroused. Sometimes both men and women are so lost in the bodily sensations of making love that they do not fantasize. This is not a better way of making love or a worse way. It is simply a different way. Sexual fantasies are not at present thought of as being essential to sexual arousal but are widely becoming recognized a means of enhancing it. The greatest domination of our sexually repressive past has probably been over the mental images of our fantasies. (Schulz 1984, 215-16)

Today, clinical sexologists encourage women to explore their sexual fantasies; and "persistently or recurrently deficient (or absent) sexual fantasies" is now a diagnostic criterion for Hypoactive Sexual Desire Disorder (DSM-IV 1994, 498), the most common sexual dysfunction in both women and men. As noted above, Kinsey mused that desire might be a factor in the incidence of SRFOs (Kinsey et al. 1953, 536).

In addition to aiding sexual desire and arousal, fantasy can be helpful in therapy. Hartmann and Fithian (1972) pioneered the use of fantasy and guided imagery to help clients remove blocks to sexual functioning in their imaginations first. For example, where there is fear of penetration on the part of a male or female, guided imagery may be used in fantasy to talk the person through the experience of penetration, orgasm, or ejaculation. Wendy Maltz and Suzie Boss, authors of *Private Thoughts: Exploring the Power of Women's Fantasies* (2001), describe the healing power of sexual fantasy for women who have experienced paralyzing physical trauma or illness. For example, women have used their imaginations to rebuild sexual desire or restore self-esteem following mastectomy.

Today, erotic books, videos, and audiotapes, designed to stimulate women's sexual fantasies, are easily available. Numerous entrepreneurs target the female population, providing both products and education. One of the leading vendors, *Good Vibrations,* has been the topic of at least one doctoral dissertation (Comella 2004). Mainstream department stores frequently offer clothing and assorted accessories to enable role-playing or dramatization of sexual fantasies. Cybersex and phone sex offer relatively safe opportunities to indulge sexual fantasies, and seem to be increasingly popular with women. Sometimes therapists even recommend sexual exploration through these media.

Kinsey found that 2 percent of the women in his sample who masturbated reported that they were able to achieve orgasm by sexual fantasy alone, without any physical stimulation (Kinsey et al. 1953, 200). One percent of Shere Hite's sample (1976) reported this ability. Wells 'found that orgasm through only fantasy or daydream (while awake) was a significant predictor of nocturnal orgasm *frequency* [emphasis mine] among women, a relationship that appears to further support the postulation that psychological stimulation is a requirement for female nocturnal orgasm" (Wells 1986, 433-4). Given the increased social acceptance of sexual fantasy for women, it is likely that a much higher percentage of women today are able to demonstrate this ability. Whipple, Ogden, and Komisaruk studied some of the physiological responses (systolic blood pressure, heart rate, pupil diameter, pain detection threshold and pain tolerance) to self-induced imagery orgasm and found that "the increases . . . were comparable in magnitude to those in the genital self-stimulation-produced orgasm condition" (Whipple, Ogden, and Komisaruk 1992, 121). The Janus survey asked women to indicate their preferred method of achieving orgasm. One percent of the female homemakers selected fantasy as their preferred method. Given that masturbation was also a choice, one might assume that this indicates fantasy without masturbation (Janus and Janus 1993, 98).

An interesting ABC *Primetime Live American Sex Survey* found a significant generation gap regarding fantasy. Among the younger respondents (ages eighteen to twenty-nine), 71 percent said they talk with their partners about sexual fantasies. This rate reduced sharply with age, averaging only 36 percent above age forty (ABC News 2005, 8).

Today, the wide variety of sexual fantasies makes it difficult if not impossible to categorize them or put them in any priority. Nonetheless, many try. Maltz and Boss (2001) separate sexual fantasies into two broad categories: *scripted fantasies*, which may contain plots and identifiable characters; and *unscripted fantasies*, which tend to focus on sensations rather than character roles. These are not mutually exclusive, though, and many women include both elements in their fantasies.

A recent Internet poll of favorite female fantasies during masturbation showed "sex with spouse/ partner behaving as usual" leading the count at 15 percent (QueenDom.com). This is one of Kinsey's categories ("thinking of the sexual relations that [one] had previously had") and is essentially reviving the memory of a pleasurable experience. Many writers seem to distinguish between memories of actual events, and imaginary events that have never transpired, counting only the latter as fantasy. Nevertheless, *remembering* is probably the most common kind of fantasy for most people (Birch and Ruberg 2000). Sometimes the memory of an experience from a dream provides the content of a waking fantasy. As author and retired sex therapist Robert Birch points out,

> Most fantasies are just private thoughts that need not have a complex storyline, or a cast of hundreds. Working too hard at building a sexual fantasy can become a distraction, defeating one of its purposes. The best fantasies are often quite simple and tied in with pleasant memories. Often it is visual, creating a mental image of a part of the partner's body that is pleasing to look at, but

impossible to see in the dark or in a particular position. At times words can be added to the fantasy while forming the mental image: "I love your buns." (Birch 2005)

Beyond these simple memories and imaginings are numerous sexual fantasies incorporating less probable events. But as David Schulz points out,

> In order to use fantasies as a means of enriching your sexual life, it is necessary to be able to understand and respect the boundary between the real world and fantasy land. Apparently fantasies are most effective when they are not lived out. Fantasists who do not live out their fantasies do not feel guilty about entertaining such thoughts in their mind. (Schulz 1984, 204)

The most popular female fantasies in 1984, as summarized by Schulz, were: imaginary lovers (often movie stars and fictional heroes), sex with more than one member of the opposite sex, forcing someone to have sex, being forced to have sex, having sex with someone of one's own gender, being handled roughly, dominance, rape or other aggression (Schulz 1984, 205-215).

Similar themes are still popular in recent polls, although today's fantasies also reflect changes in the larger culture. *Sex with a co-worker* topped one recent poll of women (Lamberti 2005). Fantasies of being photographed or videotaped seem to be popular currently, as are fantasies that allow women to play more dominating sexual roles. Nonetheless, "rape fantasies" still top the list in other polls. Aside from these, a quick consolidation of various "top ten" polls reveals the following kinds of fantasy activity: sex with a close friend, sex with a total stranger, role-playing with a spouse/ partner, playing with sex toys, sex with a movie star or musician, using objects other than sex toys, sex with a hooker/gigolo/stripper, group sex, being sexually displayed before an audience, surrendering to a master's demands, being a prostitute or lap dancer, being tied up or tying someone else up, sex with another woman.

The *Sex on Campus* survey (1997) asked about favorite sexual fantasies during masturbation. The most frequent fantasies for young women (aside from various locations) in order, were: a threesome, bondage, using a video camera, taken photographs, sex with a much older partner, an orgy, same-sex sex (if hetero), talking dirty, role-playing, S/M, sex with violence, spanking, rape, golden showers, phone sex, online sex, cross-dressing, sex with an animal, opposite-sex sex (if gay), or other (Elliot and Brantley 1997, 21). The partners about whom the respondents fantasized during masturbation were, in order: their current partner, someone they knew, no one, a celebrity, a made-up person, a stranger (Elliot and Brantley 1997, 28). Fantasies during intercourse were also surveyed. For women, sex with a friend, another lover, or an "ex" topped the list of fantasized partners; followed by celebrities, with Brad Pitt being the favorite fantasy lover (Elliot and Brantley 1997, 18).

Interestingly, Brad Pitt still tops the list in polls of college women (*Playboy*, October 2005, 105).

While clinicians today do not generally interpret sexual fantasies as evidence of pathology, they recognize that an individual's preferred fantasies often provide relief from traumatic memories or potentially inhibitory self-concept and emotional patterns (Stoller 1979). For example, fantasies can be used as "antidotes" to guilt, worry, shame or rejection (Bader 2002). Problems can arise when fantasies are too rigid, or obsessive, or lead to dangerous paraphilias or violent behaviors.

Sexual fantasy is a mental activity that requires an ability to focus attention sufficiently so that the mind can associate ideas and images with pleasurable sensations in the body. Fantasy requires both imagination, and memory of real or vicarious events associated in some way with pleasure, relief of pain or distress, or more generalized excitement. Often these associations are rather indirect (Bader 2002). While there is a tendency to think of fantasy as visual imagery, it is usually more powerful when all of the senses are included: sounds, smells, dialogue or vocalizations, sensations, and of course, emotional feelings. Many people find fantasy more effective when there is a story line or *scene*, in addition to attention on specific sexual acts.

There are numerous socialization factors which impede sexual fantasy, and some of these are certainly found in higher education. Paradoxically, some of these restrictive socialization messages ultimately provide the greatest erotic power (Morin 1995).

In any event, if more women are actively fantasizing about sex while awake, it becomes more likely that sexual imagery and feelings will surface during sleep, either as a re-shuffling of daytime experiences (continuous), *or* as a context in which to allow other repressed or unresolved material to surface (compensatory).

Anxiety and Arousal

In the surveys mentioned in Chapter Two, both *anxiety* (Winokur, Guze, and Pfeiffer 1959; Henton 1976; Wells 1986) and *arousal* (Kinsey et al. 1953; Henton 1976; Wells 1986) were correlated with SRFOs. That "sexual excitement during sleeping hours and a high degree of anxiety were positively related" (Henton 1976, 245) was the strongest conclusion of the Henton survey, with both of these conditions more prevalent among senior year college women. Over the years, the relationship between anxiety and sexual arousal has been debated. In recent years, researchers have more widely recognized that anxiety may have a facilitative effect on sexual arousal. Before reviewing studies regarding this relationship, it is probably useful to note that many sexual fantasies mentioned in the preceding section include situations that might be considered anxiety provoking. The difference is simply the cognitive interpretation or mental context.

Kinsey (1953) very astutely noted the physiological similarities between a variety of emotional states and sexual arousal. He listed fifteen elements of gross physiological sexual response which depend on the autonomic nervous system, and concluded that "the physiology of human sexual response depends only to a minimum degree upon the more highly evolved human brain" (Kinsey et al. 1953, 703). He also noted that of twenty-four sympathetic and parasympathic elements of physiological sexual response, most can also appear during states of anger, fear, or epilepsy. Male ejaculation was included in this list; however, female orgasm was not (Kinsey et al. 1953, 704). Nonetheless, other researchers have recognized "anger orgasms" and "stress orgasms" in women (Heiman, 1976). According to Kinsey, "one might hypothesize that if certain of the physiologic elements were prevented from developing in a sexual response, or taken away from a sexual response, the individual might be left in a state of anger or fear...The fact that frustrated sexual responses so readily turn into anger and rage might thus be explained" (Kinsey et al. 1953, 704). He also noted that occasionally anger or fear develop into a true sexual response.

Since the 1970s, most sex therapists have viewed anxiety as one of the most significant barriers to sexual arousal. This came from the work of Masters and Johnson (1970), and their emphasis on sensate focus exercises and other anxiety-reduction techniques.

Helen Singer Kaplan echoed this opinion, viewing anxiety as a leading cause of inhibited physiological sexual arousal through the disruption of autonomic nervous system functioning (Kaplan 1974, 125-36). Most clinicians can easily identify situations in which anxiety plays an inhibitory role in the sexual response cycle. However, the overall effect is more complex.

Jack Morin, author of *The Erotic Mind*, developed the erotic equation: "Attraction + Obstacles = Excitement" (Morin 1995, 48-71). He describes anxiety as a paradoxical aphrodisiac on both the emotional and physiological levels:

> The relationship between anxiety and eroticism is intricate and paradoxical. If you are highly anxious in a sexual situation, your physical capacities for arousal or orgasm or both will usually be short-circuited . . . However, to view anxiety solely as antithetical to arousal is to blind ourselves to a richer and more challenging reality: just as surely as anxiety can disrupt arousal, it can also create, focus, and intensify it. Depending on the situation and the individuals involved, anxiety is either an antiaphrodisiac or an aphrodisiac – occasionally both.
>
> Anxiety ntensifies arousal by contributing to a generalized state of physical excitation. All forms of excitement, sexual and nonsexual alike, increase muscular tension, blood flow, and heart and breathing rates. Consequently, your body responds similarly to anxiety-provoking and sexually arousing situations. For instance, some men and women spontaneously experience sexual arousal in a wide range of frightening situations, including everything from fights to roller-coaster rices to sexual assaults. (Morin 1995, 117-8)

In Morin's view, anxiety is inherently part of the four cornerstones of eroticism: 1) Longing and anticipation; 2) Violating prohibitions; 3) Searching for power; and 4) Overcoming ambivalence. In addition, the principle physical sensations associated with *limerence*, or falling in love, as identified by Dorothy Tennov (1979), are virtually identical to those associated with anxiety. Many of the thoughts and feelings are as well.

In 1977, Hoon, Wincze and Hoon conducted an important study demonstrating "that sexual arousal is enhanced in sexually functional women when they are exposed to an anxiety-evoking rather than relaxation-inducing film stimulus before exposure to sexual stimuli. Investigations with sexually functional men have also demonstrated a facilitatory effect of anxiety on sexual arousal . . . (Dutton & Aron, 1974)" (as summarized in Palace and Gorzalka 1990, 404). Later studies compared the relationship between anxiety and sexual arousal in both sexually functional and dysfunctional subjects. Barlow (1986) found that anxiety (threat) diverted the cognitive focus on erotic cues and altered cognitive erotic interpretations for dysfunctional men, thus inhibiting sexual arousal; whereas, anxiety (threat) actually increased the sexual response of functional men.

Palace and Gorzalka (1990) found that "anxiety preexposure enhanced the rate and magnitude of genital arousal for both dysfunctional and functional subjects [women] in relation to the

136

neutral condition. Despite increased genital responses, both groups reported less subjective sexual arousal after anxiety preexposure. Functional subjects exhibited greater physiological but not subjective arousal than dysfunctional subjects in both conditions" (Palace and Gorzalka 1990, 403). There were several other important observations in this study. Interestingly, "100% of the dysfunctional sample [n=16] experienced enhanced genital arousal after exposure to the anxiety-eliciting stimulus," regardless of symptom diagnosis. Secondly, the incongruity between physiological arousal (VBV measurements) and subjective ratings of arousal were evident in this study as they have been in almost all studies of female sexual arousal. In addition, much like Kinsey, Palace and Gorzalka hypothesized that "physiologically, 'anxiety' may enhance sexual arousal in both sexually functional and dysfunctional women because of generalized sympathetic activation that directly provides a jump start or preparedness for sexual arousal. When sexual cues are provided, this enhanced sympathetic responsivity may activate specific genital responses" (Palace and Gorzalka 1990, 408). The authors proposed that sexual arousal for women "may consist of two components: (a) a biological predisposition for physiological arousal (response lability) and (b) a conditioned cognitive expectancy for sexual arousal" (Palace and Gorzalka 1990, 408).

Cindy Meston, professor of clinical psychology at the University of Texas at Austin, has conducted several interesting studies which further explore Palace and Gorzalka's findings, and aspects of female sexual arousal in general. A series of studies with Gorzalka showed that activation of the sympathetic nervous system through twenty minutes of physical exercise (stationary bicycle) prepared, or primed, most women's bodies for greater sexual arousal in response to erotic stimuli (Meston and Gorzalka 1995, 1996a, 1996b). This was true for sexually functional women and those diagnosed with low sexual desire. "Among anorgasmic women, exercise significantly *decreased* [emphasis added] VPA but had no effect on VBV responses to an erotic film. Acute exercise had no significant effect on the women's perceptions of sexual arousal" (Meston and Gorzalka 1996a, 582).

Another study, cleverly titled *Love at First Fright* (Meston and Frohlich 2003), showed that the physiological excitement of a roller coaster ride increased subjects' ratings of attractiveness and dating desirability of opposite sex, nonromantic seatmates and opposite sex images in photographs. Variations on this experimental model are continuing.

> Excitation transfer theory, as first described by Zillman (1971), posits residual excitement from a previous arousing stimulus or situation may serve to intensify a later emotional state . . . Sympathetic nervous system arousal does not terminate abruptly with the cessation of the eliciting conditions, but . . . declines slowly . . . It is during this period of residual excitement that an individual who is exposed to a subsequent emotion-provoking situation may misattribute the residual excitement to their current situation. By doing so, their

experience of the subsequent emotional state may be intensified. (Meston and Frohlich 2003, 537)

This *excitation transfer* of anxious arousal was also noted in a recent study of heterosexual men (Bancroft et al. 2003). Although excitation transfer theory has been studied in relationship to sexual arousal since the 1970s, it seems to be receiving more attention, especially in regard to real-life settings.

Meston's lab has also recently published results from an investigation of hierarchical linear modeling (HLM) as a tool for analyzing the correlation between physiological arousal and subjective reports of sexual arousal (Rellini et al. 2005).

> Previous research indicates that women may estimate their sexual arousal according to cues other than changes in genital blood flow. Several areas of research have provided evidence for the notion that women may attend to external stimulus information as opposed to internal physiological states to determine their level of sexual arousal . . .
>
> We propose that a more appropriate way to analyze the relationship between vaginal pulse amplitude and subjective sexual arousal is to continuously and simultaneously measure the two variables throughout exposure to sexual and nonsexual films and to utilize hierarchical linear modeling for the statistical analysis. (Rellini et al. 2005, 117-118)

This approach did yield much higher intra-subject correlations between subjective and physiological arousal measurements than is common. The researchers concluded that "vaginal pulse amplitude was found to significantly predict levels of subjective sexual arousal in sexually healthy women and the inverse relationship was also true" (Rellini et al. 2005, 123). The study also raises several questions. While much of this study relates to statistical methods, the researchers developed a new device called an "arousometer" to "measure subjective sexual arousal continuously and simultaneously." One question is simply, what is the arousometer actually measuring? Comparison with Likert scale questionnaires suggested that "the arousometer was detecting changes specific to mental sexual arousal rather than affect or physiological sexual arousal" (Rellini et al. 2005, 123). Inter-subject responses were interesting. It appeared that the more sexually experienced subjects showed greater correlation between VPA and subjective reports.

> The natural question that follows from this study will involve investigating what moderates the strength of the relationship between subjective and physiological sexual arousal. Given that some women seem to have a much stronger association between physiological and subjective sexual arousal than others, it is important to understand the individual differences that may explain this variance. (Rellini et al. 2005, 123)

Since the arousometer requires real-time reporting, it would seem to be potentially useful in biofeedback style awareness training. Meston was quoted in an *APA Monitor* article commenting that, "An open question is whether the resulting sex differences in the [perception of the] relationship between physiological and subjective arousal are permanent, or whether they can be changed through training" (Meston, in Benson 2003). This would also seem to be a fruitful direction for future research.

Meanwhile, numerous female sexuality researchers, including Meston, have proposed a revised and expanded DSM classification system for female sexual dysfunction, which acknowledges the separation between subjective and physiological arousal reactions. As proposed, this would include: "Subjective Sexual Arousal Disorder," "Combined Genital and Subjective Arousal Disorder," "Genital Sexual Arousal Disorder," and "Persistent Sexual Arousal Disorder" (Basson et al. 2001; Basson et al. 2004).

Several researchers have investigated the possibility of using classical conditioning to evoke sexual arousal in women under laboratory conditions (Letourneau and O'Donohue 1997). The only study to show a positive result so far also revealed an interesting (and somewhat humorous) effect relative to the relationship between anxiety and arousal. While both men and women showed increased sexual arousal to the conditioned stimulus (CS) when it was presented subliminally, female "skin conductance responses indicated more general arousal to the [irrelevant CS, in this case a] gun than to the male abdomen" (Hoffmann, Janssen, and Turner 2004, 63).

It is important to remember that the physiology of sexual arousal is quite different than the physiology of orgasm. Increasingly, it also appears that the brain responses of female arousal and orgasm are quite different than male brain responses. For example, in one fMRI study, the amygdala (sometimes considered to be part of the temporal lobes) and hypothalamus were shown to be more active for men during sexual arousal than for women, although most brain regions showed similar activation patterns (Hamann et al. 2004). Activation of the amygdala is also associated with fear, anxiety, and emotion. For many years, primarily as a result of brain disease and brain lesion studies, the amygdales have been recognized as playing an important role in sexual arousal (Rhawn 1996, Chapter 4, for summary). In the Holstege et al., PET studies (2003, 2005), the amygdales of both men and women were virtually deactivated during orgasm. As more data is gathered through brain imaging technology, it is possible that new models of the human sexual response cycle will emerge.

In summary, it is likely that both sexual arousal and anxiety are highly correlated with SRFOs, because they are often related to each other. Fortunately, this relationship is receiving more attention by researchers. Since the hypothalamus directs the activity of the autonomic nervous system, which includes the sympathetic and parasympathetic arousal responses, and is also responsible for regulating system homoeostasis, it would be natural to assume that the inhibition provided by sleep would facilitate resolution of this sympathetic arousal through orgasm. As previously noted in Chapter Three, Masters, Johnson, and Kolodny suggest that this is true for both men and women, though no specific mechanism is hypothesized:

> If there has been considerable excitement but orgasm has not occurred . . . there is sometimes a lingering sensation of pelvic heaviness or aching that is due to continued vasocongestion. This may create a condition of some discomfort, particularly if high levels of arousal were prolonged. Testicular aching ("blue balls") in men and pelvic congestion in women may be relieved by orgasms that occur during sleep. (Masters, Johnson, and Kolodny 1982, 76)

One question arising through this discussion is the extent to which *excitation transfer of anxious arousal* contributes to sexual dream content and SRFOs. The possibility of this transfer, combined with the activation of the hypothalamus during arousal, suggests that SRFOs may indeed play a compensatory role in regulating system homeostasis in a very broad way, not necessarily due to discharge of *sexual energy* per se.

Another set of interesting questions comes from the relationship between high education/career activity (versus homemaking) and anxiety. Do highly educated career women experience greater anxiety? If so, are they choosing to interpret it as sexual arousal? Have they developed a "conditioned cognitive expectancy for sexual arousal" (Palace and Gorzalka 1990)? Are they choosing orgasm as an anxiety management tool, consciously through masturbation and unconsciously through SRFOs?

Conversely, to what extent do women interpret sexual arousal as anxiety, especially during the premenstrual phase? Given the difficulty that most women demonstrate in subjectively recognizing sexual arousal as such, this misinterpretation is an obvious possibility. Both men and women will benefit greatly from increased awareness of excitation transfer mechanisms and sexual arousal cues. Further research and education on this topic will be greatly appreciated.

CHAPTER 7: SPIRITUAL, RELIGIOUS, SOCIAL, AND POLITICAL CONSIDERATIONS REGARDING SRFOs

Overview

Many today might consider SRFOs to be a simple biological reflex, triggered perhaps by random brain activity, active dream-state imagination, or unresolved arousal. Throughout history, however, this response has been intimately interwoven with belief systems regarding humanity's relationship with spirits, demons, god(s), and immortality, as well as belief systems about the relationship between men and women. While religious doctrines have significantly shaped political control of conscious sexual behavior, at times both religious and political policies have even more vigorously viewed erotic dreams, and sleep-related orgasms and emissions, as their special domain.

Kinsey paid special attention to the role of religious attitudes in his investigation of SRFOs.

> The number of females in the sample who had ever experienced nocturnal dreams to the point of orgasm (the accumulative incidence), and the number who were having such experience within a five-year period (the active incidence), did seem to have been affected by the degree of their religious devotion . . .
>
> The differences were not dependent on the Protestant, Catholic, or Jewish backgrounds, but upon the degree of

their devotion in their religion. In general, fewer of the females who were active or devout religiously had dreamed to the point of orgasm – perhaps because they had had the smallest amount of overt sexual experience about which they could dream. . .

On the other hand, the frequencies with which the females had had dreams after they had once started them did not seem to be affected by the religious background . . . It will be recalled that we found a similar situation in regard to the masturbatory frequencies of the females in the sample . . . It is difficult to understand why a religious background which has kept a female from dreaming of sex for some period of years does not continue to influence her after she has begun to have sex dreams. (Kinsey et al. 1953, 203-5)

It would appear from Kinsey's data that a change in *attitude* (discussed in Chapter Six) might have affected the rate of SRFOs and masturbation among this group.

As discussed in Chapter Two, the *compensatory* theory had been popularized since the beginning of the twentieth century, resulting in both Catholic and Jewish codes recognizing nocturnal dreams as "the only acceptable form of sexual outlet . . . outside of vaginal coitus," and only under strict conditions (Kinsey et al. 1953, 207). For the most part, these *acceptable* conditions required a total lack of voluntary control or consent, combined with passive disgust. "Such dreams are without fault or sin provided that (1) they are not deliberately induced by thought or deed; (2) they are not consciously welcomed and enjoyed" (Kinsey et al. 1953, 207). Catholic theologians described in detail the kinds of thoughts and behaviors, before, during, and after sleep-related sexual experiences, that were deemed to be sinful or sin-free (Arregui 1927, 6; Davis, 1946, 243; as reported in Kinsey et al. 1953, 207). "The Jewish interpretation is typified by the statement in Leviticus 15:15-16, that nocturnal emissions make one unclean, and one must wash and be unclean until the evening" (Kinsey et al. 1953, 208). The language and behavioral descriptions in these statements do not directly acknowledge *female* sleep-related orgasms. "The moral significance of nocturnal sex dreams has most frequently been considered in connection with the male, but the principle has, on occasion, been extended to the female" (Kinsey et al. 1953, 208).

The notion of compensatory value was also used by the Catholic church and others "to contend that there are no biologic or medical reasons which should make it impossible for anyone, female or male, to remain completely abstinent and chaste before marriage" (Kinsey et al. 1953, 208) or in any other condition. As mentioned in Chapter Two, Kinsey's data did not generally support the compensatory theory either in frequency or circumstance (Kinsey et al. 1953, 211). Overall, "the average frequencies for those [women] who were having [orgasmic] dreams . . . remained around 3 to 4 times per year from adolescence to the oldest age groups . . .at least to age sixty-five" (Kinsey et al. 1953, 201).

Pleasure and Volition

The current Catholic teachings emphasizing *volition*, the intentional application of will or choice, and *lack of pleasure,* have been part of the morality debate throughout history.

As traced by cultural historian Riane Eisler in her book *Sacred Pleasure: Sex, Myth, and the Politics of the Body* (1995), the societal view of sexual pleasure as sinful started to develop during the Bronze Age (between 4000 and 2000 B.C) as part of a process to separate men from women, and develop men as cold, compassionless warriors. This period saw the rise of war gods (like Yaweh), the cultural institution of women as property (domestication), the shift to patrilineal bloodlines, and the "dehumanization of men" (Eisler 1995, 120).

In most Western civilizations under the influence of the Judeo-Christian teachings, sexual pleasure under any circumstances has been viewed as sinful because it selfishly glorifies the body or carnal nature rather than sanctifying the Spirit and placing the relationship with Christ at the forefront. Current Catholic teachings emphasize that standards for sexuality within marriage (the only acceptable framework) must "preserve the full sense of mutual self-giving and human procreation in the context of true love" (*Humana Persona*, 1975, Section V). There is no specific mention of pleasure.

Nonetheless, as noted by Kinsey and others, women report enjoying the vicarious and physical pleasure of erotic dreams and SRFOs more than men, and simply accept them with less worry or moral distress (Kinsey et al. 1953, 214).

The issue of volition is more complex, due to the relative unconsciousness of sleep. St. Augustine, in the fifth century, was the first Christian writer to specifically address the topic of morality in sleep. His conversion "from a philandering pagan to an ascetic Christian" (Flanagan 2000, 18) occurred in his early thirties, and he frequently experienced erotic dreams. In his autobiographical *Confessions*, he addressed this question to God:

> You commanded me not to commit fornication . . . But when I dream [thoughts of fornication] not only give me pleasure but are very much like acquiescence to the act . . .Yet the difference between waking and sleeping is so great [that] I return to a clear conscience when I wake and realize that, because of this difference, I am not responsible for the act, although I am sorry that by some means or other it happened in me. (Augustine circa 397, in Flanagan 2000, 18)

Augustine concluded that dreams are *happenings* rather than actions, and are therefore not sinful. "Whereas one is responsible for what one does or chooses to think about, one is not responsible for thoughts that involuntarily occur in one's mind" (Flanagan 2000, 18). Nonetheless, Augustine did recount other people's dreams which seemed to be lucid and volitional within the dream. While

Augustine is frequently mentioned today, his position regarding lack of responsibility for nocturnal emissions has not been consistent church policy throughout the years, as will be discussed further below.

It is probably important to note that there are three points at which one might exercise volition, and therefore accrue responsibility: before, during or after the event. One might exercise will before sleep with the intention of inducing (or denying) an erotic dream or sexual experience. Likewise, following such an occurrence, one can choose to interpret or assign meaning to the experience. Owen Flanagan, author of *Dreaming Souls* (2000) comments specifically on the morality of volition within the dream:

> Augustine is right that committing adultery, murder, and so on in dreams normally is not sinful. However, given a certain conception of morality, it may be possible to be immoral while dreaming. Many traditions hold us accountable for our thoughts and characters as well as our actions. On the view I'll be defending, dreams are sometimes, and to varying degrees, identity expressive. To the extent that the shape of our characters is under voluntary control and deformed, then we may express certain bad aspects of ourselves when we dream. Some evidence suggests that for certain individuals - primarily lucid dreamers, that is dreamers who know they are dreaming while they are — the plot and content of specific dreams can fall under executive control. If morality is tied to choice and control, then it follows that for such dreamers, their dreams may reasonably be judged as morally revealing, and thus they are to some degree responsible for what they dream about. (Flanagan 2000, 19-20)

The current standards (volition and pleasure) actually represent a rather *enlightened* perspective on this topic compared to those which preceded them. These standards began to emerge around 1760 (Stewart 2002), due to scholarly discussion by doctors and others. In the eyes of the Christian churches, for over three hundred years immediately prior to that time, erotic dreams and sleep-related orgasms and emissions were usually considered to be the result of interaction with the incubi (male) or succubi (female) demons, satanic devils, or fallen angels. In fact, by the fourteenth century, dreaming itself had become sinful and dangerous, regardless of the subject matter, because of the potential influence by demons (Van de Castle 1994, 82). Charles Stewart of the Royal British Anthropological Institute, in a research paper on *Erotic Dreams and Nightmares from Antiquity to the Present*, reports that between 1650 and 1850 there were at least twenty-five articles published regarding this topic (Stewart 2002), and since two treatises published in 1760 (Jaccard 1975, 11), erotic dreams, emissions and orgasms have been separated from nightmares and demonic interaction and

> placed in a separate category centering on masturbation
> . . . Erotic dreams involved a form of mental
> masturbation, *delectatio morosa*, and became a subject
> for the emergent discipline of sexology (Ellis, 1936
> [1898]) . . . In this period, the term 'incubus' went from

denoting an independent demonic being to denoting an objective set of physical conditions . . . Physical and medical explanations naturalized both the erotic dream and the nightmare, although there was still sporadic support for the idea that external spirits produced dreams. (Stewart 2002, 20)

Under this enlightened view, even allowing the possibility of volition, nocturnal emissions and SRFOs would be no more morally damaging than masturbation.   Realistically however, since the eighteenth century there have continued to be both moral and medical condemnations of masturbation (Hall 1992). The sin of Onanism became a disease, as described by Tissot in 1758; and male nocturnal emissions became the disease of spermatorrhea (Wong 2002, 264). Most of the literature from this period relates to men, and a variety of devices and medical procedures were designed to eliminate erections during sleep. Yet "onanism was often seen as the cause of many disorders that plagued nineteenth century women . . . and any unexplained ailment could potentially be accused of onanism . . . hysteria, in particular" (Wong 2002, 265). When healthy living (diet, exercise, fresh air) did not produce cures, a few medical procedures, such as "application of carbolic acid to the clitoris and electroshock therapy . . . and for the most stubborn cases, . . . clitoridectomy" (Wong 2002, 265) were used to deter female masturbation.

The work of Kinsey, Masters and Johnson, and many others in the field of sexology during the last half of the twentieth century significantly shifted personal *and* public attitudes regarding masturbation, as discussed in Chapter Four. Nonetheless, 50 percent of the respondents in the NHSLS (Michael et al. 1994, 166) reported feelings of guilt about masturbation. In the mid 1990s, when Jocelyn Elders, Surgeon General of the U.S. Public Health Service, suggested teaching masturbation in sex education classes, there was public outrage based on *moral* and religious grounds. Today, a quick Internet search produces numerous articles by many different religious groups still condemning masturbation on moral grounds, and in some cases, spreading erroneous health information. The official position of the Catholic Church today as expressed in *Persona Humana* (1975), is that "every genital act must be within the framework of marriage" (Section VII); and that

> whatever the force of certain arguments of a biological and philosophical nature, which have sometimes been used by theologians, in fact both the Magisterium of the Church – in the course of a constant tradition – and the moral sense of the faithful have declared without hesitation that masturbation is an intrinsically and seriously disordered act. (*Persona Humana* 1975, Section IX)

This document further states that, depending upon the circumstances, masturbation can be a *mortal* sin. While it addresses a range of issues related to sexuality and chastity, there is no specific mention of nocturnal emissions or sleep-related orgasms.

In some communities, there has been heated debate about how and what to tell boys in sex education classes about nocturnal emissions or *wet dreams* (Kempner 2003). And as noted in the introduction to this paper, female sleep-related orgasms are not included in sex education classes at all.

Spiritual Issues Unique to Women

When compared to the discussion regarding nocturnal emissions for men and boys over the past 250 years, there has been relative silence regarding SRFOs. In reviewing the literature, it becomes apparent that these sleep responses in women have historically been viewed quite differently than the sleep responses of men. It is important to note that at the time of Kinsey's report, there still existed deeply rooted spiritual fears regarding sleep-related orgasms. In the early years of the Christian church, debates about volition in dreams, character development, and morality really applied only to men. Since the Bronze Age, in most of western civilization it has been assumed that women were so physically, mentally, and spiritually defective that they did not even have the ability to exercise volition in support of moral development. The cultural perceptions of women assumed that they were inherently unable to be in control of their thoughts, will, and sexual appetites

154

under any circumstances (Dean-Jones 1992). Both Judaism and Christianity were formed as misogynistic, male-ruled religions. While "the Orthodox Jewish man thanked God every morning that he wasn't born a woman" (Sjoo and Mor 1987, 292), the Christian St. Clement commented that "every woman should be overwhelmed with shame at the very thought that she is a woman" (in Sjoo and Mor 1987, 292). It was not until the Ecumenical Council at Macon in A.D. 900, that with a one-vote margin, it was decided that women even have souls, with the deciding vote cast by a radical bishop of the Celtic church (Sjoo and Mor 1987, 292).

> Both Old Testament and Christian priests saw physical love as the archenemy of the spirit; it was Anti-Christ, it was Satan – female snares lining their path to the disembodied hereafter. Long before Freud, the cosmic serpent was reified into a "bestial" symbol of sexual love. Counseled that women were the "tempters" – unclean deceivers of the male soul – young boys were trained to be constantly on guard, even in dreams against "female wiles" . . . This training in sexual paranoia was all-pervasive in Christendom; without it, the Inquisition could never have happened. (Sjoo and Mor 1987, 289)

While much of this attitude came from the Biblical story of Eve, and assorted teachings of the war gods and their priests, it was also reflected and reinforced by early medical assessments. Hippocrates, for example, was of the opinion that a woman's migrating womb would sometimes move to her head and could "stifle those organs in which consciousness was thought to lie" (Dean-Jones 1992, 78).

Overall, *female* sleep-related orgasms, more than the emissions of men, have provided a point of convergence for several major fears that have plagued Western civilization for the past 5,000 years. These fears, all created and maintained by religious teachings, are: 1) fear of the spiritually ecstatic, life-bearing power of female sexuality; 2) fear of sexual pleasure in general; 3) fear of the power of dreams to access spirit worlds; and 4) fear of sexually-assaulting, potentially impregnating spirits. While the first two fears have dominated waking sexuality, the last two have been almost exclusively associated with sexuality in sleep. And while this latter fear may seem strange to many twenty-first century Americans, it is really as old as human civilization. Teachings of the newly vocal and organized Christian fundamentalist groups are reviving these old fears and concerns. For example, the first response to *The Good Wife* blog (2005), Appendix A, raises concerns about demons. Another web site, www.demonbusters.com, mentions a contemporary female Christian evangelist who teaches that nine out of ten women are sexually attacked by demons in their sleep, often without their knowledge. This message is also being delivered from pulpits and in classrooms. Some of the scientific responses to this belief will be discussed later in this chapter. At this point, however, it is useful to recognize that this is not a *dead* belief, and it appears to be part of the reason why SRFOs are not publicly discussed. One British researcher reports that

> There is still a strong belief in the reality of supernatural beings that are able to have sex with humans. In fact, there are probably more reported cases of supernatural sexual assault today than there ever were during the height of the witch trials and, unlike the tortured confessions of the witches, these stories are given voluntarily. (Deane 2003, 44)

The idea that there exist spiritual beings capable of having sex with humans seems to be a basic belief in almost all human religions and mythologies throughout time, East, West, North or South. This belief was a basic premise associated with the Inquisition and consequent witch-burnings. "The history of witch burning is pivotal to an understanding of Western history" (Eisler 1995, 413); and it is likewise pivotal to an understanding of female sexuality, *especially* Sleep-Related Female Orgasms. Given that the lack of discussion of SRFOs today may be, at least to some degree, based on the same fears that propelled the actions of the Inquisitors, public discussion of SRFOs is likely to bring forth these deep cultural beliefs, fears and prejudices. On the other hand, it might provide an opportunity for twenty-first century humanity to move into an enhanced understanding of spirit, self *and* sexuality. Therefore, an understanding of the moral issues related to SRFOs requires a brief historical review.

Judaism

In the Jewish tradition, nocturnal emissions had been considered a source of spiritual *pollution* since the early books of the *Old Testament*, written around 800 B.C. As noted in Chapter Five, the *Old Testament* of the *Bible* contains numerous stories of dreams, many of which include contact with life-transforming spiritual guidance. The Jewish *Talmud*, a collection of sixty-three volumes of rabbinical literature connecting the *Old Testament* from around 500 B.C. to the Greco-Roman period around A.D. 300, contains 217 references to dreams, expressing many different viewpoints, including the "belief that supernatural entities such as evil spirits, demons, and the returning dead could instigate dreams" (Van de Castle 1994, 52). The Jewish scholars also acknowledged that good entities, such as angels, could be the sources of dreams and thereby deliver messages to mortals. They also recognized soul travel in dreams. However, most dreams were thought to be the result of everyday events: emotions, food, weather conditions, occupation, and other mundane experiences. Nonetheless, the overall attitude was the statement from Rabbi Hisda, who said, "An uninterpreted dream is like an unread letter" (in Van de Castle 1994, 54). The Jewish tradition does not appear to address volition within dreams; however, there is a long tradition of prayers before sleep to influence dream experiences. As noted also, the emphasis on dream interpretation implies volition following the dream. There are no dreams by women recorded in the *Bible*, the *Talmud,* or in any of the near Eastern cultures of that time, with the exception of the Egyptian records (Van de Castle 1994, 54).

The *Talmud* also includes references to *Lilith* as the primary instigator of erotic dreams. She was also mentioned in the Jewish *Midrash* or folktale tradition, the *Dead Sea Scrolls*, and the Sumerian tablets before these. Her full story was not recorded until the *Alphabet of Ben Sira,* written anonymously between the eighth and tenth century A.D., and elaborated more fully in the twelfth century *Kabbalah,* and *Zohar.* Briefly, Lilith was the first wife of biblical Adam, created in the same manner as he was. Adam and Lilith fought over many issues; and eventually she left him to live in the spirit worlds, by pronouncing the "Ineffable name" (*Zohar*, 3:76). She was particularly angry that he never let her be on top during sex. Because she left before the fall from the garden, she retained her immortality, and birthed hundreds of spirit children each day. Two conflicting lines in the *Bible* support her existence. In the first chapter it states that "So God created man in his own image, in the image of God he created him; *male and female* [emphasis mine] created he them" (Gen. 1:27). In the next chapter Adam is alone, and God creates Eve from his rib (Gen. 2:21-22). There are many traditions attributed to Lilith, and in modern days she has become a heroine to many feminist groups. In the early days of the *Talmud*, she was most well known for inducing men to have ejaculations during sleep so that she could steal their semen to become pregnant. According to the Kabbalah, her male offspring have the ability to impregnate human women (*Zohar* 3:76). The cover of darkness, and unconsciousness of sleep have provided the primary conditions under which this occurs. Nocturnal emissions and orgasms have often been used as evidence of these unions.

The non-physical perpetrators have variously been viewed as gods, demons or nuisances; and likewise, their offspring have been viewed as saviors and royalty, demons and witches, or miscreants. For example, in addition to Jesus, there were sixteen slain savior-gods believed to have lived and died for the sins of the world between Osiris in Egypt, 1700 B.C., and Mithra in Persia, 400 B.C. (Bushby 2001, 196). According to legends, most were born of virgins or some sort of spiritual insemination. Many other historical and mythological personages were also thought to have been conceived by union with non-physical spirits, including Alexander the Great (according to Plutarch), Merlin, Caesar Augustus, the father of William the Conqueror, Plato, and Martin Luther (Hyde 2005). Likewise, for many centuries, children with birth defects were considered products of these unions.

The Greco-Roman Influence

Spiritually, the Egyptian, Greek and Roman scholars of the pre-Christian period were not as concerned about sexual demons during sleep as were the Mesopotamians. Although they recognized a variety of such spirits (*ephialtes,* in Greek), usually associated with nature and other gods like Pan or Diana, they placed more emphasis on communication with guiding spirits, or the use of dreams to receive or discern the gods' mandate for human actions.

For at least a thousand years before the Christian church, dream incubation was used widely as a primary healing and spiritual tool, in civilizations from Greece through China and India. This would imply some degree of volition expressed before the dream, and some degree of volition expressed in the interpretation that follows the dream. During that period, there were many dreaming temples; and the abilities to interpret dreams, or to dream information for another, were highly valued skills of the oracles. In addition, Plato for example, emphasized the use of dreams for character development, as an opportunity to demonstrate that the rational mind and spirit can tame the appetitive desires (Stewart 2002). This would imply volition during the dream. Nevertheless, at that time among the Greeks, volition within dreams seemed to apply only to men, due to the perceived mental defects of women.

Women were sometimes valued as dreamers, and more rarely as interpreters of dreams. They also served as channels for guidance from the spirit worlds. During the thousand years before Christianity, there were ten major oracles or centers of prophecy in the ancient worlds (Monaghan 1997). The Oracle at Delphi (Greek), named Pythia, was active from 1400 B.C. to fourth century A.D. and respected worldwide. Various female priestesses filled the role of Pithya's mouthpiece. The nearby Temple of Apollo served as a frequent gathering place for scholars. The Cumaean Sibyl, near Naples, served the Roman Emperors. Many of her prophecies were bound into books and consulted for a thousand years, until the sixth century A.D. According to legend, she was physically immortal due to an agreement with Apollo. Constantine consulted with her before battles, and referred to her prophecies before and during the Council of Nicaea in 325 A.D. The *Sibylline Books* were considered sacred texts. Constantine used these prophecies to derive his authority to create a new gospel for the masses (Bushby 2001, 216). These prophecies were last publicly consulted by Emperor Justinian at the Fifth Ecumenical Council of 553, held in Constantinople, where the Roman Church banned the Druidic and Essene doctrines related to reincarnation, as well as many other long-held beliefs about the nature of the soul (Bushby 2001, 223). With the rising power of Christianity, the oracles and their prophecies formally became heresy, and the spiritual misogyny of the Judeo-Christian philosophy suppressed women even further.

For the pre-Christian Greeks and Romans, it was recognized that the meaning of sexual dreams was often symbolic and unrelated to sex. For example, for a man to dream of sex with his mother usually meant good fortune, especially for politicians (Stewart, 2002,

162

7). Conversely, dreams with no overt sexual content could be related to sex or pregnancy. Erotic dreams and nocturnal emissions were not a moral issue, although emissions were briefly considered to be a health concern. The Greek doctors and scholars had significant influence throughout the Hellenistic and later Roman empires. However, given the large variety of belief systems during this period, their teachings and values were not universally accepted. The Epicureans of Rome, for example, assigned no value whatsoever to dreams (Van de Castle 1994, 77).

The Christian Influence

The early Christians, especially Tertullian of Carthage (160-202 A.D.), placed great value on dreams, especially as a source of revelation. In his *Treatise on the Soul*, which devoted eight chapters to his study of sleep and dreams, Tertullian proclaimed that dreaming was evidence of the soul's immortality and its attribute of *ekstasis,* the ability to stand outside of the mortal life events. He also argued that people were not responsible for the events that transpired in dreams, and saw the ability to remember dreams as a special gift. Although he acknowledged the role of demons in producing some dreams, he felt that even these "sometimes turn out to be true and favorable to us" (Kelsey 1968, 245). His views were popular among some Christian groups for over a thousand years (Van de Castle 1994, 77-78).

After Christianity was formally instituted at the Council of Nicaea in A.D. 325, the topic of erotic dreams became a moral issue, primarily for the Christian ascetics, since according to the Judeo-Christian philosophy, sexual pleasure was sinful as were women in general. While the new Christian church did not require celibacy (some early priest were married), it did require chastity or continence even if married, and male priests were not allowed to live under the same roof with their wives.

The next writer to have a significant impact regarding the morality of dreams was Jerome, who was born into a Christian family in the fourth century, after Christianity became the official state religion. He was a student of the *Bible*, but read extensively in the Greek and Latin pagan classics. At one point, when he was distressed about his inability to reconcile conflicting teachings, he experienced a profound clarifying dream and for a period "went into the desert as a hermit" (Van de Castle 1994, 79). Although he was a flamboyant transvestite whose "dress became the origin of cardinal's garb today" (Bushby 2001, 173), he became a great Bible scholar, and in A.D. 382 he was called to Rome to translate the entire Bible into Latin.

> His translation, later known as the Vulgate, served as the authoritative Latin version of the Bible until the twentieth century. This literary event had a cataclysmic effect upon how dreams were viewed by western Christians for the next fifteen centuries. Jerome apparently deliberately mistranslated the Hebrew word for witchcraft, *anan*, which was considered a pagan

superstitious practice, as (*observo somnia*), "observing dreams." The word *anan* appeared ten times in the Old Testament; seven times Jerome correctly interpreted it, as witchcraft or a closely related practice, such as divining; but in the other three cases, where the Hebrew text is specifically condemning witchcraft (*anan*), he redirected the condemnation against dreams (Kelsey, 1968, p. 159). Thus, the prohibition "you shall not practice augury or witchcraft" became "you shall not practice augury nor observe dreams." Since he had correctly interpreted *anan* seven times, Jerome was clearly aware of the word's accepted meaning . . .

It's possible that the change was ordered by church officials, but Jerome may also have had personal reasons for his mistranslation . . . [He] may have sought to shore up his defenses against his pagan impulses . . .

Jerome's mistranslations changed the course of Christian belief and practice regarding dreams [emphasis mine] . . . This link between dreams and forbidden practices had its main effect in the Latin-speaking western Christian church; the favorable view toward dreams in the eastern Christian church, which followed the Greek Bible, was not significantly altered. (Van de Castle 1994, 79-80)

This policy relates to volition after a dream, the choice to not *observe* it, interpret it, believe it, or give it any meaning. The condemnation of dreams was an effective tool for limiting direct spiritual revelation and making the populace more dependent on ruling priests for spiritual guidance. It also allowed dream insights to be condemned as witchcraft, and provoked a deep fear of dreaming.

It took several centuries for the impact of Jerome's interpretation to be felt by the public, since at the time of his translation the church was new and most of the Roman Empire was pagan. Initially, these teachings had their greatest impact on those who were actively involved in the Church hierarchy (monks, priests, ascetics, etc.). Eventually, however, the results of this translation error were felt by all of western civilization (Stewart 2002; Van de Castle 1994).

Macrobius, a fourth century contemporary of Jerome's, wrote a book called *Commentary on the Dream of Scipio*, which was the first Christian publication to discuss the existence and activities of demons, the incubi and succubi, who sexually-assaulted humans during sleep. This book became very popular and influential, with thirty-seven printed editions before 1700.

> It was the most important and well-known dream book in medieval Europe. Its inclusion of the fear-inspiring sexual demons was to play a role in supporting the paranoia about evil spirits that developed during the later centuries. (Van de Castle 1994, 80)

Augustine, writing in the fifth century, also discussed the incubi and succubi in his influential book, *The City of God* (circa 413). He was convinced of their existence, and acknowledged that they "have often injured women, both by desiring them and acting carnally with them" (in Deane 2003, 32). He considered them more as nuisances than evil, and included "the sylvans and fawns," as well as the *Duses* of Gaul as incubi. He did not hold humans responsible for these contacts (Deane 2003, 32).

Throughout the first ten centuries of Christianity, "girls were generally not deemed to have been at fault if they had been taken advantage of by a demon or angel, and so there can be little doubt that some unplanned pregnancies were blamed on supernatural forces" (Deane 2003, 45). This gradually changed between the thirteenth and fifteenth centuries. This was probably due in part to the Church's concerns about declining influence and the rising protestant movements. The Crusades were having an "ideological side-effect: Returning feudal lords brought back 'exotic' religious and lifestyle ideas (including the Tantric sexual arts) from the 'lands of the infidels'" (Sjoo and Mor 1987, 298-9). The Church began to emphasize the role of Satan and devils in prompting disobedience and dissension, as well as causing plagues and wars. Since dreams had long been recognized as doorways to spirit worlds, dreams were viewed as a primary opportunity for satanic influence and the introduction of heretical thoughts.

By the eleventh and twelfth centuries, issues regarding volition in dreams were surfacing. St. Thomas Aquinas, writing in the thirteenth century, also emphasized the opportunities for satanic influences during sleep and dreams, and consequently fueled some of this. "The first witch to be executed for copulating with a demon was put to death in 1275, one year after the death of Saint Thomas

Aquinas, a Doctor of the Church, whose contribution to the witch-incubus belief was considerable" (Masters, R.E.L. 1966, xiii-iv). Church leaders began to view the nocturnal demons as much more evil, and humans as much more responsible for attracting or inviting them.

Standards that previously applied only to the male ascetics or clergy were being applied to the population at large. Pre-sleep prayers and rituals became common. Starting around 1200 A.D., people were being officially killed as "heretics" (Sjoo and Mor 1987, 298). By the fourteenth century or so, it was not only considered sinful for the common man to examine or believe dream content, but even to dream at all. "Aside from belief in them, dreaming itself had now become a hazardous nocturnal activity . . . Dreaming became something people tried actively to suppress" (Van de Castle 1994, 84).

> [There was a] shift in theological dogma that gained a general acceptance after 1400. According to this revised position, the Church had been correct in its early teaching that incubi and succubi exist and have intercourse with humans. However, the demons of the early Christian period forced their attentions upon humans – in other words, committed rapes. But after 1400, the intercourse of demons with humans took a new and sinister turn. Witches appeared in great number, and for the first time the intercourse with demons was voluntary on the part of the humans engaging in that gravest of sins. (Masters 1966, xiv-xv)

By this time, many people, including those in emerging Protestant movements, were genuinely afraid of the satanic influences.

> In 1484, therefore, Pope Innocent VIII pronounced a Papal Bull against the now-suddenly-discovered crime of *witchcraft*. He denounced witchcraft as an organized conspiracy of the Devil's army against the peace and common order of the Holy Christian Empire (a peace and common order which people living under that empire had rarely experienced). And thus the war against women was officially launched by the Christian papacy, as a diversionary tactic to keep itself in power through the strategy of sheer terror. (Sjoo and Mor 1987, 299-300)

In 1486, with papal blessings, two Dominican monks, Heinrich Kramer and Jakob Sprenger published a book called *Malleus Maleficarum*, or the *Witches' Hammer*, and for the next three hundred years this church document was used to authorize the torture, imprisonment, and deaths of perhaps hundreds of thousands of people, throughout Europe, western Asia, and even the new world colonies including South America. Some estimates place this death toll as high as nine million including those who died in prison (Sjoo and Mor 1987).

This lengthy and extremely misogynistic document is organized into three parts with many sections in each part, describing in detail the ways in which witches (always assumed to be women) might be identified; how they operated; how they should be

169

made to confess; and how to punish them. "Sexual intercourse of humans with devils was the central fact of witchcraft" (Masters 1966). "There are sexual elements in all the signs of sorcery that are advocated. A common practice was to look for strange marks or moles on the thigh or breast, which were thought to have been put there by the devil . . . Other sexual signs were confessions of having had sex with the demons known as succubi and incubi" (Deane 2003, 79). Repeatedly the *Malleus* declared that human females were inherently the agents and tools of the Devil. Part I, Question Six, details dozens of reasons why this was so, and a few excerpts are included from multiple paragraphs:

> All wickedness is but little to the wickedness of women . . . . What else is a woman but a foe to friendship, an unescapable punishment, a necessary evil, a natural temptation, a desirable calamity, a domestic danger, a delectable detriment, an evil of nature, painted with fair colours . . . They are more credulous; and since the chief aim of the devil is to corrupt faith, therefore he attacks them . . . [they] are more impressionable, and more ready to receive the influence of a disembodied spirit . . . they have slippery tongues . . . women are intellectually like children . . . she is more carnal than a man, as is clear from her many carnal abominations . . . The word woman is used to mean the lust of the flesh . . . The many lusts of men lead them into one sin, but the one lust of women leads them into all sins . . . When a woman thinks alone, she thinks evil . . . All witchcraft comes from carnal lust, which is in women insatiable . . . Wherefore for the sake of fulfilling their lusts they consort even with devils. (Kramer and Sprenger 1971[1486], 41-47)

Regarding punishment (Part III), the authors essentially concluded that because of women's nature, exorcism was ineffective. In addition, "Christian exorcists were effective only with Christian demons – because of their ritual, which was the only one they were permitted to use - serious problems could occur if a foreign or pagan devil possessed a Christian" (Masters 1966, 109). Therefore, it was deemed that the only alternative, for the benefit of society and the witches' immortal souls, was to kill them after torturing them to obtain a confession. The injunction from Exodus 22:18, "Thou shalt not suffer a witch to live," was used as Biblical justification. Conversely, when a man was "defamed" by being accused of heresy or sexual interaction with devils, he could receive a "canonical purgation" by denying the charges under oath and producing "*men* [emphasis mine] of his own station and condition" to vouch for his "his habits" (Kramer and Sprenger 1971[1486], 241-42). Surveys following this period of history estimate that 72 percent of all those accused of witchcraft were women, and in some areas this figure was as high as 92 percent. Only in Russia were slightly more men than women accused of sorcery (Levack 1992).

> The difference between the first ascetics and the laity during the witch craze was that earlier a (male) individual had largely been left to monitor his own spiritual failures. Later (male) clerics decided this matter on behalf of (female) individuals. Torture and capital punishment replaced internally imposed humility and renewed ascetic effort as responses to erotic dreams. (Stewart 2002, 18)

At that time it was deemed that women were approximately nine times more likely than men to experience these demonic sexual liaisons, due to the much higher number of male demons, combined with women's insatiable lust, inherent spiritual defectiveness, and total inability to resist any sexual advances. And yet women were held morally accountable.

> The inquiring authorities . . . assumed that witchcraft must involve sexual acts with the Devil and thus they pushed the stories in that direction through questioning. Judges showed a particular interest in the issue of whether the intercourse with the devil was voluntary or forced, frightening or pleasurable (Kramer & Sprenger 1970 [1486]:114; Lancre 1982 [1613]: 200-1). Whether or not actual erotic nightmares or erotic dreams had occurred to the accused, there was a likelihood that erotic nightmare scenarios would occupy a conspicuous place in the final confession. (Stewart 2002, 18)

Realistically, there were other charges as well which resulted in death. Witches were accused of causing male impotence, castration, sex changes, sterility, miscarriage, and other sex related problems. Various forms of herbal or spiritual healing were deemed to be witchcraft. Midwives were thought to play key roles in arranging incubus liaisons, killing babies, and creating infertility. Older, post-menopausal women were more commonly accused of witchcraft due to their supposed need for the life force of male semen. In addition, homosexuals and non-Christian pagans were considered to be under demonic influence. Non-Christians were deemed the equivalent of animals, so sex with a non-Christian human was a form of beastiality, also enumerated as an activity of the Devil (Deane 2003, 83). "It seems rather odd that Christian lawgivers should have adopted the Jewish code against sexual intercourse with beasts, and then enlarged it so as to include the Jews themselves" (Evans 1906, 157).

Given that the witch-hunts sometimes resulted in residents of entire towns being executed with all properties going to the Church, it is likely that the true motivation for the witch burnings, especially in the later years, had more to do with acquiring wealth than saving souls (Sjoo and Mor 1987).

To a very great extent, the evidence for witchcraft was based on sexual experiences during *sleep, with or without awareness.* At that time, it was common for several people to sleep in the same room or even the same bed. Records from witch trials show that during this period, there was often great confusion among both women and some inquisitors as to whether or not any of the sexual deeds really happened, or were products of imagination or dreams. Several writers of that period debated this point to no avail, while other writers debated the roles of drugs, sexual frustration, sleep walking, suggestibility, mental disorder, etc. (Masters 1966). Overall, many of these questions and issues were never really resolved (Steward 2002). One of the most comprehensive discussions of the psychology of this period is R.E.L. Masters' book, *Eros and Evil: The Sexual Psychopathology of Witchcraft* (1966), which includes the complete text of Fr. Ludovico Maria Sinistrari's late seventeenth century classic treatise on *Demoniality.*

There are many different theories as to why the witch trials eventually ended. Finally, for whatever reasons, more men started questioning, writing, and speaking out against the practice in the eighteenth century. Nonetheless, witch burnings were a daily occurrence during the seventeenth century (Sjoo and Mor 1987, 302), and continued sporadically through parts of Europe much longer. The last witch burning occurred in Peru in 1888; and many witches were executed by lynching through "the nineteenth century: in Germany, 1836; in France, 1850; in England, 1863" (Masters 1966, xiv). The last witch trial in England, which ended with a successful prosecution, took place in 1944, as Great Britain was preparing to enter WWII (Deane 2003, 93).

Current Trends and Relevant Research

Spirit Sex

As stated prior to the historical review, it should not be surprising if fear of demons surfaces in present day discussions of SRFOs. Twenty-first century America has a fascination with the supernatural, as evidenced by prime time television shows (*Medium, Ghost Whisperer*, etc.), magazines, and the Internet. In addition to the admonitions expressed by Christian fundamentalists, almost every Internet discussion of dreams, which this writer has accessed, includes cautions about demons.

On the other hand, the Internet is also filled with more pleasurable orgasmic accounts of sex with *ghosts*, extra-terrestrials, incubi, succubi, angels, spirit guides, Jesus, the Holy Spirit, assorted energy presences, and other supernatural beings. One can even find detailed instructions for how to cultivate on-going orgasmic sexual liaisons with incubi and succubi partners. Some of the reported experiences are induced. Some reports indicate spontaneous occurrences during sleep, dreams, relaxation, meditation or prayer. For some, these are sexual adventures that could be considered an emerging fantasy genre. For some women these are deeply emotional, nurturing contacts. And still other women report profoundly spiritual, life-changing experiences. It is beyond the scope of this paper to assess the reality of these contacts; however, there is no doubt that from the subjective perspective of the reporters, these experiences are fulfilling a need or desire.

Among Christian ascetics today, especially Catholic nuns, there is a growing movement toward recognizing "sexuality – erotic energy – as a powerful sacred fire" (Weingarten 2005, 61).

> For Sandra Lommasson, 56, opening spiritually took a
> different form. "I had a sense of God coming to kiss me

with an open mouth. I didn't know what to do with that because I wanted God on my terms, and that felt terribly intimate . . . "

"The Juice" is how Sister Lorita Moffatt, on the Mercy Center staff, described sexual energy. "It's the juice of life, a desire for union, communion, and it's in plants, animals, and all of creation. Consider The Juice as The Holy Spirit inviting us into close relationship with God and with other human beings." (Weingarten 2005, 61)

This should not be surprising for several reasons. Throughout history there have been reported outbreaks of "erotomania" in Catholic convents throughout the world (Masters 1966, 104-110). However, the more important reality is that for the first 200,000 years of human life, culture and *spirituality* were dominated by the mysteries of the female body (Gadon 1989). *Woman's spiritual practice was naturally ecstatic, orgasmic, and somewhat trance-like, fusing the sexual and the spiritual as one.* "In the original religion of the Great Mother, body and mind and spirit are always integrated" (Sjoo and Mor 1987, 53).

Despite these pleasurable life-enhancing reports, there still exist many present-day accounts of frightening visitations and nighttime abductions by non-physical beings, which are neither pleasurable nor orgasmic, although they often have sexual content or overtones. As Stewart comments, "The popular cultivation of orgasmic dreams today would seem to suggest the end of the erotic nightmare, but the matter is not so simple. Recent developments suggest that the erotic nightmare might be headed for a more mainstream revival" (Stewart 2002, 26).   In recent years, several lines of scientific inquiry have begun to shed light on these occurrences.

The Sensed Presence

The sustained belief in supernatural night visitors comes not only from religious *teachings,* but also, from the actual *experiences* that people have reported throughout time, across all cultures. Experiential reports of sleep related assaults by spectral beings have never been *un*common.   Cross-culturally, these experiences have been called by many names, including nightmares, the "old hag" experience, and the "night crusher."   Increasingly scientists are using the term, *sensed presence* (Cheyne 2001) or *feeling of presence (FOP)* (Conesa 2000) to acknowledge not only the visual hallucination, but also the interactive *feeling* of these experiences. Researchers from many fields have begun to explore this phenomenon.

Anthropologist David Hufford, now at Penn State College of Medicine, was the first to make the connection between these reports and the sleep disorder known as *sleep paralysis (SP)* (Hufford 1976). He was studying folklore in Newfoundland in 1971 when he first heard tales of the "old hag." Typically, sleepers reported waking up being physically paralyzed with an evil presence or old witch on top of them creating strong pressure on their chest, and thus creating a feeling of inhibited breathing. While there were slight variations in the reports, they were often terrifying. After a few seconds or minutes, the *old hag* would leave and movement would be restored. Further investigation revealed that this has been a relatively common experience in many cultures throughout time, including those that had never heard of witches or incubi.

> This sensation of presence is one of several features . . . typical of what sleep researchers call sleep paralysis, and that comprise a remarkably complex pattern found all over the world. A pattern that sounds like a folktale, a story from a pre-modern society where evil spirits are a part of daily conversation, but a pattern that turns out to be equally common in nineteenth century Boston and twentieth century Seattle. (Hufford 2005, 5)

The word nightmare actually comes "from Anglo-Saxon *merran,* meaning to crush. The term eventually morphed into nightmare – the crusher who comes in the night" (Bower 2005, 2). Although different cultures would use terms that fit their cultural beliefs and myths, the experience would be essentially the same. Hufford's book, *The Terror that Comes in the Night*, was published in 1982, and many writers and researchers have addressed this topic since then.

Sleep Paralysis, noted by Dement and considered originally to be a symptom of narcolepsy, is an anomalous REM state condition that "consists of a period of inability to perform voluntary movements either at sleep onset (called hypnogogic or predormital form) or upon awakening (called hypnopompic or postdormital form)" (Demert 1999). Today it is recognized as a separate disorder, and when it occurs in the absence of any other condition, it is often referred to as Isolated SP (ISP). In the predormital form, the brain bypasses the NREM stages of the sleep cycle. As explained in Chapter Three, during REM sleep the brainstem turns off the sleeper's motor abilities and much sensory input. In sleep paralysis, this happens while the sleeper is still conscious or awake, and often able to open eyes. In some ways, the postdormital form is actually just opposite of SRFOs, in which the body's sensory/motor abilities appear to be partially returning while awareness is still in the dream or sleep. However, this might not always be the case, since female orgasms do not require motor abilities as shown by Holstege's PET scan research (2005); and they do occur *during* the REM stage as shown by LaBerge's research (1983).

Sleep researchers often refer to the SP condition as a "hiccup" in the brain wave cycle, a minor glitch that lasts only a few seconds or minutes. No one is known to have ever died from SP; but the subjective experience might feel like impending death (Dement 1999). ISP is often accompanied by very clear visual, auditory, kinesthetic/ tactile, and spatial hallucinations that co-exist with the sleeper's ability to clearly perceive the room in which they're sleeping. The perception of "pressure or pushing on the body may be so intense that the person feels as though s/he is being pushed or pulled into the bed" (Cheyne 2001, 146).

> In some cases, when the hypnogogic hallucinations are present, people feel that someone is in the room with them, some experience the feeling that someone or something is sitting on their chest and they feel impending death and suffocation. That has been called the "Hag Phenomena" and has been happening to people over the centuries. These things cause people much anxiety and terror, but there is no physical harm. (Dement 1999)

However, the hallucinations are not *only* terrifying. In some cases they are experienced simultaneously as both terrifying and profoundly spiritual. For some, they have constituted a spiritual awakening with life-changing insights. They are compelling, yet not delusional (Cheyne 2001). "The sense of presence considered here is an 'other' that is radically different from, and hence more than a mere projection of the self. Such a numinous sense of otherness may constitute a primordial core consciousness of the animate and sentient in the world around us" (Cheyne 2001, 136). Some people who experience SP frequently can train themselves to convert these experiences into lucid dreams or more pleasurable encounters (Conesa 2000).

Consciousness researchers and neurophysiologists have been busily trying to discern the mechanisms that allow the brain to create such perceptions. Whalen (1998) suggests that they arise from a "vigilance system" involving several limbic structures including the extended amygdala, the nucleus basalis of Meynert in the substantia innominata, and the anterior cingulated cortex system.

Research suggests that a disposition toward ISP is definitely familial (Conesa 2000), although it might be a function of nurture rather than genetics. It seems to be more prevalent in China, parts of Africa, and among those of African descent. In international samples, between six and sixteen percent of respondents report an SP experience at some time in their life (Conesa, 2002). In studies to date, this figure is as high as 44 percent among Nigerian nursing students, and 39 percent among African-Americans. Among Americans and Japanese overall, the rate of SP reports is around 22 percent. It is higher in some occupational groups. Various studies have shown that it might be related to lack of sleep, psychological or physical stress, anxiety, depression, occupation, developmental changes (especially in the age eighteen through twenty-seven period), geographical location, or ecological conditions such as electromagnetic fields due to technology or earthquakes (Conesa 2000, other studies summarized in Conesa 2004, 38-44). One study "found that 35% of subjects with ISP also reported a history of awake panic attacks unrelated to the experience of paralysis" (Dement 1999). "In severe cases, where episodes take place at least once a week for 6 months, medication may be used" (Dement 1999). Drug therapy typically includes antidepressants such as imipramine. Most recommendations for treating SP suggest basic good sleep hygiene; i.e., get plenty of rest, avoid stress, exercise moderately but not immediately before sleep, and unique to this condition, avoid sleeping in a supine position (on one's back).

Jorge Conesa, an ecopsychologist and sleep researcher, currently in the Department of Neurology of the University Hospital of Berne, Switzerland, conducted a ten-year longitudinal case study of SP and its relationship to a variety of factors including types of dreams. The study ran from 1992 to 2002, and included 5,761 dream events associated with the ISP condition. The results were published in a 2002 journal article, and a 2004 book, *Wrestling with Ghosts*, which will be republished in an expanded revision in 2006. He responded to this writer's email inquiry regarding whether it is possible for women to experience orgasms during SP. His response:

> NO. However, because, as you know, the transition between SP and lucid dreams (when orgasms are reported) can be swift, it is easy to conjoin these two events, phenomenologically, so that it seems that the orgasm happened during an SP episode.
>
> For example, a person can experience an SP event first, then move to a dream (REM) where they are laying down and where they dream that sexual intercourse is imminent and acceptable, then experience an orgasm, and finally move out of the REM phase into SP again. This sequence can later be remembered and re-told as SP being a central experience during orgasm. Moving in and out of these stages and cycles is very dynamic making a

phenomenological evaluation of these subjective states confusing and challenging.

In short, the SP event is usually a terrifying one, thus it is antithetical to sexual enjoyment or orgasms. (Conesa, personal email, October 30, 2005)

Michael Persinger of Laurentian University has been researching *The Neuropsychological Base of God Beliefs* (1987) since 1971. To date he has published over 200 journal articles and six books. In recent years he has focused on the impact of weak electromagnetic field patterns on neural synapses. Such stimulation of the temporal lobes has led to the experience of the *sensed presence* phenomenon and other paranormal perceptions during *wakefulness.* In the lab he uses a "helmet" to generate specific field patterns and field effects. However, Persinger contends that people are exposed to these daily in a variety of ways, including proximity to electrical power lines and geo-physical events like earthquakes. Many consider his work to be quite controversial, to the extent that it might be interpreted as a denial of God. Nonetheless, it is a relevant piece of the consciousness puzzle. He responds to this criticism in the following way:

The research is not to demean anyone's religious/mystical experience but instead to determine which portions of the brain or its electromagnetic pattern generate the experience. Two thousand years of philosophy have taught us that attempting to prove or disprove realities may never have discrete verbal (linguistic) solutions because of the limitation of this measurement. The research has been encouraged by the historical fact that most wars and group degradations are coupled implicitly to god beliefs and to the presumptions that those who do not believe the same as the experient are somehow less human and hence expendable. Although these egocentric propensities may have had adaptive significance, their utility for the species' future may be questionable. (Persinger 2000)

In recent years, many researchers have attributed a variety of paranormal and spiritual experiences to the sensed presence phenomenon, usually as it occurs in sleep paralysis, since so many reports are associated with sleep or relaxation. Currently this seems to be a significant component of the scientific explanations for UFO abduction experiences (Stewart 2002; Conesa 2004; Clancy 2005), as well as incubi/succubi contacts (Hufford 1982; Cheyne, 2001; Deane 2003; Conesa 2004; and others). Therefore, it is important for sexologists to be aware of this research. (Many consider reported alien/ET contacts to be simply a modern, culture-based interpretation of the SP experience.)

On the other hand, even among scientists there is acknowledgment that this is not the final answer. A recent paper by Hufford (2005) explores this and concludes that sleep paralysis *is* a genuine spiritual experience, though obviously subject to a variety of interpretations.

It is because the majority of SP experiences include the perception of apparently incorporeal beings that I have called them spiritual experiences. And this is the reason that the response of so many experiencers is spiritual or religious, as I will show. *Spiritual experience* also refers to experiences interpreted by the subject in a manner that points to a spirit. In the modern western world this is most acceptable when the spirit referenced is either God or one's soul. The dramatic spiritual experiences that elicit strong negative sanctions are those that involve the apparent perception of a spirit, that is, those closest to the old, core meaning of *spiritual.* The resut has been the remarkably effective suppression of reporting of SP and the consequent underestimation of its prevalence . . . (Hufford 2005, 18)

The modern explanation that the contents of such experiences are internally generated fantasies comes up short in the face of the consistency of independent experiences. (Hufford 2005, 41)

Overall, it appears that current knowledge does not *fully* explain the content of reported sleep paralysis experiences, or the reactions of those who experience them. The burst of research in recent years is generating interesting data, discussion, hypotheses, and perspectives.

CHAPTER 8: SUMMARY AND RECOMMENDATIONS

The topic of Sleep-Related Female Orgasms has been neglected in recent years and merits far more research and public awareness. A large, unknown percentage of women experience these orgasms. If trends from previous research have continued, the present day incidence might exceed 50 percent among mature women. This experience almost always occurs quite spontaneously, often with awareness of a dream. Although it is frequently experienced as quite pleasurable, there is sometimes resulting confusion due to a lack of accurate, professional information in the public domain. Men, including many who treat women in a variety of professional settings, are likewise confused and uninformed. Nonetheless, SRFOs appear to be neither unhealthy nor rare.

As Kinsey noted, it appears that there is no single factor, or cluster of factors, that is predictive of SRFOs in an individual history; and different factors can act in different ways at different times even for the same individual (Kinsey et al. 1953, 212).

This paper suggests that overall, sleep mentations are more continuous than compensatory; therefore, sexual content and experience during sleep would be more likely among women who think about sex when awake. These cognitions include memory, fantasy, desire, imagination, prosexual attitudes, knowledge of SRFOs, and familiarity/safety with sexual pleasure and the orgasmic reflex. It is likely that formal education, intelligence, personality characteristics, and other cultural factors influence these sleep mentations. Orgasmic responses during sleep seem more likely when there is some level of autonomic nervous system arousal before sleep, including both psychological and physiological elements. Physiological elements include lingering arousal from waking orgasms or sexual behavior during partnered sex, masturbation, or active fantasy. Arousal may also be due to hormonal fluctuations, physical exercise, or emotional states such as anxiety, or anger. In these latter cases, SRFOs might serve a compensatory role in maintaining system homeostasis. It is likely that SRFOs occur more frequently among lucid dreamers due to possible neurological conditions unique to the lucid dream state, and the conscious freedom to exercise volition by choosing pleasure.

Research is somewhat hampered by the very large number of possible variables related to this response, and the multi-disciplinary nature of the context in which the response occurs. These issues have been discussed at length throughout this paper. While the topic lies clearly within the field of sexology, little has been done to advance understanding since the dedicated research of Kinsey et al. (1953). The most notable addition was the work by Barbara Wells (1986), which highlighted the impact of cultural variables. Sleep researchers, neurophysiologists, neuropsychologists, dream researchers, and anthropologists have also made significant contributions since Kinsey's time.

Data Gathering and Possible Research Hypotheses

Over the past fifty years, there have been changes in some of the psychological, behavioral, and cultural factors suspected to have an impact on SRFOs. One could easily hypothesize, therefore, that there have likewise been changes in the incidences and frequencies of these responses. The Henton (1976) and Wells (1986) surveys support this hypothesis. A first role for sexologists, it would seem, would be to gather current data regarding incidences and frequencies. In recent years, large sexological surveys using representative samples have not inquired about this topic.

Given the *total* lack of current information, it would seem that *any* survey of contemporary women, regardless of the sample, would represent an advance over what is now known. Any sample including women above college age would be very useful since these ages have not been surveyed regarding this topic since Kinsey; and Kinsey's data suggested that incidences of these responses increase throughout the life span and might peak in the forty to fifty-five age ranges.

The Internet provides a relatively inexpensive mechanism for surveying. Surveys could be designed to test a variety of relevant hypotheses. Some of the hypotheses suggested by research in this paper include:

1. A high percentage of American women do not know that some women experience SRFOs (supported by Wells 1986).

2. Most women today have learned about SRFOs from their personal experience (not explored previously).

3. Women enjoy SRFOs (supported by anecdotal reports and Kinsey 1953).

4. Knowledge of SRFOs is, in itself, a predictor of sleep orgasms (Wells 1986).

5. Liberal attitudes toward sexuality are predictive of SRFOs (Wells 1986).

6. Formal education is a predictor of SRFOs (Unacknowledged by Kinsey 1953; supported by data from both Kinsey 1953 and Wells 1986).

7. Active incidence of SRFOs increases throughout the lifespan (not supported by Kinsey 1953).

8. Accumulated incidence of SRFOs increases throughout the lifespan (supported
   by Kinsey 1953).

9. Lucid dreaming ability is a predictor of SRFOs (reported, but not explored previously).

10. Experience with meditation and other altered-states-of-consciousness (ASC) is a predictor of SRFOs (explored previously in relation to lucid dreams, but not SRFOs).

11. Frequency of SRFOs is related to stages of normal hormonal fluctuations; i.e., menstrual cycle, pregnancy, post-partum period, menopause (not explored previously, though supported by anecdotal reports).

12. Pre-sleep sexual arousal is a predictor of SRFOs (partially supported by Kinsey 1953; and Wells 1986).

13. Pre-sleep anxiety is a predictor of SRFOs (supported by Wells, 1987, Henton 1976, and Winokur, Guze, and Pfeiffer 1959).

14. Ability to experience orgasm by fantasy alone (imaginal ability) is a predictor of SRFOs (partially supported by Wells 1986, and suggested by Kinsey 1953).

15. Frequent thinking about sex when awake is a predictor of sex dreams and SRFOs (suggested by empirical dream research).

16. Frequent waking sexual experiences, including masturbation and multiple orgasms, are predictors of SRFOs (supported by Kinsey 1953; not supported by Wells 1986).

17. Desire for sexual experience is a predictor of SRFOs (suggested by Kinsey 1953).

18. Loss of previously active sexual outlets is a predictor of SRFOs (partially supported by Kinsey 1953).

19. Both high and low levels of satisfaction with sex life are predictors of SRFOs (partially supported by Kinsey 1953, and Wells 1986).

20. There are significant cross-cultural variations in the incidence and frequency rates of SRFOs (not previously explored, but suggested by Wells 1986 data).

21. Pre-sleep physical exercise is a predictor of SRFOs (not previously explored, but supported in part by excitation transfer theory).

Some of the hypotheses mentioned above require more than a respondent's subjective opinion or recollection for substantive conclusions. Nonetheless, surveys would provide useful baseline data. In addition to hypotheses amenable to survey research, there are several other research hypotheses suggested by information in this paper which require training, testing, and/or therapeutic intervention:

22. Pre-sleep sexual arousal, combined with desire and intention, can be used to induce SRFOs (suggested by some, not previously explored).

23. Hypnos s and/or self-hypnosis can be used to induce SRFOs (suggested by some, not previously explored).

24. Induced SRFOs can be a useful treatment for sexual dysfunctions (suggested by LaBerge 1990, in the case of lucid dreaming).

25. Assertive, creative and/or self-directing personality factors are predictors of SRFOs (partially suggested by Maslow 1942, and others).

26. Intelligence is a predictor of SRFOs (not previously explored).

27. Certain sleep disorders (i.e., narcolepsy, sleep paralysis) are correlated with SRFOs (not previously explored).

Further research in neurophysiology, neuropsychology, sleep, dreaming, consciousness, and anthropology will also continue to expand understanding of SRFOs.

Public Awareness

This paper has summarized what is known about SRFOs based on existing research. It is assumed that as more information becomes available to researchers and clinicians, it will eventually surface in the public domain. Certainly, far more contemporary research and data gathering are needed.

This paper began, however, with a simple question in this writer's mind, "Why don't more people know that women can, and do, experience sleep-related orgasms?" Some of the answers have included 1) lack of inclusion in sex education classes; 2) lack of contemporary research; 3) lack of public discussion; and 4) historical association with powerful fear-based religious beliefs.

The next question becomes, "Is there a need for the public to be more aware of SRFOs?" Support for this need is based on the following:

1. Many women are experiencing these orgasms and unable to find appropriate, accurate information (See Appendix A). In the absence of accurate information, a wide range of inaccurate information surfaces, including fear-inspiring notions.

2. This wr ter has had numerous recent conversations with licensed, educated health professionals of both sexes who have indicated that the idea of female orgasms during sleep is a totally new (and in some cases, shocking) revelation. Some women have mentioned SRFOs to their therapists or other health care providers only to be told that they had "never heard of such a thing."

3. In recent conversations, more than a few women have mentioned that they never in their lives have discussed this topic with anyone (spouses, girlfriends, etc.), despite their life-long experience of SRFOs. In some cases this silence has been prompted by women's concerns that there might be

something "wrong" or "abnormal" about themselves as in examples #5 and #7 of Chapter One.

4. In recent conversations, a surprising number of women have mentioned that they have "never heard of such a thing." The most common initial response from these women is a blank stare followed by a question like, "How would I know if I ever experienced one of those?" Once informed, in some cases, there has been a trace of concern about *not* having ever experienced an SRFO.

5. Some girls experience their very first orgasm as an SRFO (5 percent in Kinsey et al. 1953), which could be even more confusing than it is for older women.

What then, are the best mechanisms for increasing public awareness? It is this writer's opinion that both female and male sleep-related orgasms should be discussed in sex education classes. This includes providing girls with a proper name for these experiences, other than *wet dreams*. This paper suggests the designation of *Sleep-Related Female Orgasm* (SRFO), since *nocturnal orgasm* is inaccurate. Of course, the obvious differences between male and female responses; i.e., less frequent, typical later age onset, possible association with stages of menstrual cycle, etc., should be mentioned. Both boys and girls, and men and women, should understand that it is common and healthy for people to have sleep-related orgasms and emissions, with or without erotic dreams.

Aside from the need for young people to be informed, there is a need for older adults to be aware of SRFOs since onset often occurs in middle age. The topic definitely needs to be included in human sexuality continuing education courses for health care providers, beyond the occasional comment that, "Some women have these too." Perhaps SIECUS, ASSECT, The American College of Obstetricians and Gynecologists, or Planned Parenthood could be encouraged to develop a topical brochure as a model for local health departments to use in distribution to medical offices, along with the typical brochures on other sexological issues. Writers and speakers need to be able to address the issue of "sexually assaulting demons," should it surface, as well as all of the other factors addressed in this paper, especially arousal, anxiety, and loss of previous sexual outlets (divorce and widowhood).

Further investigation of SRFOs is likely to provide a greater understanding of mind-body interactions and female sexual response in general. SRFOs demonstrate the power of thought/fantasy/imagination. They also highlight the role of orgasm in maintaining healthful system homeostasis. In addition, SRFOs have significant implications for therapeutic assessment and treatment. Inquiry as to incidence of sleep-related orgasms should be included as part of any sexological diagnostic assessment for women as well as men (Hartman and Fithian 1972, 42). It is possible that the conditions of sleep and dreaming may actually provide a treatment milieu (as suggested by LaBerge 1990), free from many physiological and psychological inhibitions.

Beyond use in assessment and treatment of dysfunctions, SRFOs provide one more way for women to explore the power of their sexuality; know themselves better; and experience greater pleasure, joy, and satisfaction.

APPENDIX - A

Dream Incubation-by Gillian Holloway, PhD

(excerpted from the audio cassette Dream Incubation: Asking for the Dreams You Want)

Dream incubation is a time-honored technique dating as far back as recorded history. Simply put: it means to ask your dreams to address a certain question in your life. Learning how to ask your dreams for guidance on important life questions could be one of the most important things you ever learn. Although the technique seems to work like magic sometimes, it is not a game, and I suggest you proceed to try it with sincere interest rather than for entertainment. My clients have used incubated dreams to help clarify conflicting feelings, point out pit-falls in business, highlight tendencies that held them back, and even enhance creative productivity.

Bridge to The Subconscious

This technique works best for people who have a regular practice of remembering and recording dreams, because the basics of intrapsychic communication are already in place. However many newcomers to dreams are astounded at how easy the technique is, and how well it works. You will be speaking with a highly functioning portion of your psyche that is already engaged in sifting through the most pressing challenges and questions of your current situation. It is perfectly natural that this area of consciousness would provide useful information and perspectives when given the opportunity to do so. Be sure the thing you wish to focus on is truly important to you. This technique is most effective when there is a strong emotional or personal connection with what you are asking about.

Here is the basic step-by-step procedure for Incubating a dream:

1. **Get Clear On the Topic:** Prior to sleep go over in your mind the basic components of the issue. Don't try to solve it: instead identify the place in the road where you have gotten stuck. "I want to finish graduate school, but I can't afford childcare." "I want to take this new job, but I'm scared." Some people make notes about their process, others say a prayer, meditate, or simply go over the situation mentally. Make it a light process to delineate your position.
2. **Synthesize a Question:** Devise a single sentence asking a question about your target topic. Open-ended questions seem to work better than yes-or-no questions. Here are some good examples:
   - What is likely to happen if I take this job?
   - What can I do to help my partner be more loving?
   - What am I overlooking in my relationship with my son?
   - What is the lesson in this experience?

o   Why can't I seem to forgive?

Avoid questions you might ask the 8-Ball. They are inappropriate, and generate rather confusing dreams that leave you back where you started. Here are some examples of what not to ask:

o   Should I marry John?
o   Do I trust Al?
o   Will I get this job?
o   Is my relationship good?

3. **Repeat the question:** Repeat the question over and over in your mind while waiting to go to sleep. I often match the question with my breathing pattern, rather like a mantra, thinking half the question on the inhalation and half on the exhalation. Some people love this relaxing sensation, others find it annoying and complex. Just relax and repeat the question gently as you drift asleep.

4. **Record the dream:** You may spontaneously awaken when an incubated dream ends. I believe this is a natural response to your request for the information: you are being given an opportunity to remember the dream and transfer its content into your long term memory. The method I recommend to most people is the tag approach. Have a pad or pencil beside the bed so that you can make a note about the dream. Just use a word or even a sentence that sums up the dream for you. "My affair with Cary Grant" or "Scrubbing the Titanic." Then roll over and go back to sleep. When you awaken in the morning, the tag you stuck on the dream will act as an anchor or memory trigger for the entire dream, and then you will need to record it more fully.

Occasionally some people find that the tag approach doesn't work for them and they need to write down the entire dream when they awaken. If you keep a journal, be sure to jot down the question you asked next to the dream you had in response. If you remember several dreams from that night, you must assume they all potentially contain information about your question. Research as well as the anecdotal experience of dreamworkers indicates that separate dreams on a single night usually address the same theme or life context from different perspectives.

After you have captured the result of your incubation by recording the dream, you are ready to absorb the insight that has come to the surface. The dreams which are a product of your incubation question are likely to be quite obvious in their meaning. You may not need to do much digging into their imagery in order to understand what is being presented. However, I recommend you carefully examine your written record, even after a few days time to make sure you agree with your original assessment. In other cases, you will feel the importance of the dream, it will seem heavy with meaning for you, but you may need to unravel some clues about the dream's imagery. This then is the next step in the process:

5. **Reflect on the Dream:** Allow some time to elapse between recording the dream and attempting to understand it fully. One excellent approach is to record the dream in the morning and wait until evening to examine it's meaning. Sit down and sort through the imagery of the dream; examining the action, feelings and imagery. Although many incubated dreams have very obvious meaning, some may take longer to decipher. Share your dream with friends and let them reflect the metaphors they notice. Above all trust your own take on it. When you understand a dream you will get a tingle, a click, or a gut feeling.

Dream of the Month

REFERENCES

ABC News. 2005. *Primetime Live American sex survey*. Accessed 23 July 2005 at http://abcnews.go.com/Primetime/print?id=15621

Adams, Cecil. 1981. Do women have wet dreams? *The Straight Dope*. Chicago Reader. Accessed 18 March 2005 at www.straightdope.com/classics/al_061.html

Ahern, Geoffrey. 2005. *Behavioral neurology of lobar syndromes*. On-line course of University of Arizona Health Sciences Center: 15-27. Accessed 25 June 2005 at
    http://www.eddev.arizona.edu/courses/sbs/y2/docs/Psych-Neuro.pdf

American Academy of Pediatrics. 2001. Report of the Committee on Psychosocial Aspects of Child and Family Health, and Committee on Adolescence, Sexuality Education for Children and Adolescents. *Pediatrics* 108, no. 2:498-502.

Antrobus, John S., and Mario Bertini, eds. 1992. *The neuropsychology of sleep and dreaming*. Hillsdale, NJ: Lawrence Erlbaum Associates.

Armstrong-Hickey, D. 1991. A validation of lucid dreaming in school age children. *Lucidity* 10, no.1-2: 250-54.

Arnow, B.A., J.E. Desmond, L.L. Banner, G.H. Glover, A. Solomon, M.L. Polan, and
    S.W. Atlas. 2002. Brain activation and sexual arousal in healthy, heterosexual males. *Brain* 125:1014-23.

Arregui, A.M. 1927. *Summarium theologiae moralis, ad recentem codicem iuris cononici accommodatum*. Bilbao: El Mensajero Del Corazon de Jesus.

Aserinsky, E., and N. Kleitman. 1953. Regularly occurring periods of eye motility, and concomitant phenomena during sleep. *Science* 118:273-74.

Augustine (St. Augustine). 1993 [413]. *The city of God.* Translated by Marcus Dods. NewYork: Random House.

Augustine (St. Augustine). 1960 [397]. *Confessions of St. Augustine.* Translated by John K. Ryan. New York: Doubleday.

Bader, Michael J. 2002. *Arousal – The secret logic of sexual fantasies.* New York: St. Martin's Press.

Bakan, Paul. 1978. Dreaming, REM sleep, and the right hemisphere: A theoretical integration. *Journal of Altered States of Consciousness* 3:285-307.

Baker, R. R., and M. A. Bellis. 1995. *Human sperm, competition, copulation, masturbation, and infidelity.* London: Chapman & Hall. Baker, Robin. 1996. *Sperm wars.* New York: Basic Books.

Bancroft, John, Erick Janssen, David Strong, Lori Carnes, Zoran Vukadinovic, and J. Scott Long. 2003. The relation between mood and sexuality in heterosexual men. *Archives of Sexual Behavior* 32, no. 3:217-30.

Bancroft, J., J. Loftus, and J.S. Long. 2003. Distress about sex: A national survey of women in heterosexual relationships. *Archives of Sexual Behavior* 32, no. 3:193-208.

Barbach, Lonnie G. 1975. *For yourself: The fulfillment of female sexuality.* Garden City: Doubleday.

Barlow, David H. 1986. Causes of sexual dysfunction: The role of anxiety and cognitive interference. *Journal of Consulting and Clinical Psychology* 54:140-48.

Bass, Alan. 1994. Aspects of urethrality in women. *Psychoanalytic Quarterly* 63: 491-517.

Basson, Rosemary, and Lori A. Brotto. 2003. Sexual psychophysiology and effects of sildenafil citrate in oestrogenised women with acquired genital arousal disorder and impaired orgasm: A randomized controlled trial. *British Journal of Obstetrics and Gynaecology* 110:1014-24.

Basson, Rosemary, J. Berman, A. Burnett, L. Derogatis, D. Ferguson, and J. Fourcroy. et al., 2001. Report of the International Consensus Development Conference on Female Sexual Dysfunction: Definitions and classifications. *Journal of Sex & Marital Therapy* 27:83-94.

Basson Rosemary, S. Leiblum, L. Brotto et al. 2004. Revised definitions of women's sexual dysfunction. *Journal of Sexual Medicine* 1: 40-8.

Benson, Etienne. 2003. Sex: The science of sexual arousal. *APA Monitor on Psychology* 34, no.4, accessed on-line 24 August 2005 at: www.apa.org/monitor/apr03/arousal.html

Berman, Jennifer, and Berman, Laura. 2001. *For women only*. New York: Henry Holt and Company.

Bible (*The Oxford annotated Bible, revised standard edition*). 1962. New York: Oxford University Press.

Birch, Robert W. 2005. *Sexual fantasies: Parts 1-3*. Accessed 3 September 2005 at www.eNotalone.com

Birch, Robert W. and Cynthia L. Ruberg. 2000. *Pathways to pleasure: A woman's guide to orgasm.* New York: PEC Publishing.

Bower, Bruce. 2005. Night of the crusher. *Science News Online*. 168, no. 2 (July 9)Accessed 17 October 2005 at www.sciencenews.org

Braun, C.M.J., M. Dumont, J. Duval, I. Hamel, and L. Godbout. 2003. Opposed left and right brain hemisphere contributions to sexual drive: A multiple lesion case analysis. *Behavioural Neurology* 14, no.1-2: 55-61.

Brill, A. A., ed., 1995. *The basic writings of Sigmund Freud.* New York: The Modern Library.

Bushby, Tony. 2001. *The Bible fraud.* Hong Kong: Pacific Blue Group.

Calleja, J., R. Carpizo, and J. Berciano. 1988. Orgasmic epilepsy. *Epilepsia* 29, no. 5: 635-9.

Carlson, Robert H. 2003. Female sexual arousal disorder remains a mystery: Defining objective markers may help in treatment of anorgasmia, researchers say. *Urology Times* (November). Accessed on 18 August 2005 from www.highbeam.com

Cheyne, J. Allan. 2001. The ominous numinous. *Journal of Consciousness Studies* 8, no. 5-7:133-50.

Clancy, Susan. 2005. *Abducted: How people come to believe they were kidnapped by aliens.* Boston: Harvard University Press.

Cohen, Harvey D., Raymond C. Rosen, and Leonide Goldstein. 1976. Electroencephalographic laterality changes during human sexual orgasm. *Archives of Sexual Behavior* 5, no.3:189-99.

Cohen, D. B. 1977. Changes in REM dream content during the night: Implications for a hypothesis about changes in cerebral dominance across REM periods. *Perceptual and Motor Skills* 44:1267-77.

Comarr, A. Estin, Jeffery M. Cressy, and Michael Letch. 1983. Sleep dreams of sex among traumatic paraplegics and quadriplegics. *Sexuality and Disability* 6, no.1:25-9.

Comella, Lynn. 2004. *Selling sexual liberation: Women-owned sex toy stores and the business of social change*. Ph.D. diss., University of Massachusetts, Amherst.

Conesa, Jorge. 1995. Relationship between isolated sleep paralysis and geomagnetic influences: a case study. *Perceptual and Motor Skills* 80:1263-1273.

------. 2000. Geomagnetic, cross-cultural and occupational faces of sleep paralysis: An ecological perspective. *Sleep and Hypnosis* 2:05-111.

------. 2002. Iso ated sleep paralysis and lucid dreaming: Ten-Year longitudinal case study and related dream frequencies, types and categories. *Sleep and Hypnosis* 4, no. 4:132-142.

Conesa-Sevilla, Jorge. 2004. *Wrestling with ghosts: A personal and scientific account of sleep paralysis.* Pennsylvania: Xlibris Press. Forthcoming 2006. New York: Random House.

Dane, J., and R. Van de Castle. 1991. A comparison of waking instructions and posthypnotic suggestion for lucid dream induction. *Lucidity* 10, no. 1-2:209-14.

Davis, H. 1946. *Moral and pastoral theology*. Vol. 2: Commandments of God. Precepts of the church. New York: Sheed and Ward.

Davis, Katharine B. 1929. *Factors in the sex life of twenty-two hundred women*. New York: Harper & Brothers.

Dean-Jones, L. 1992. The politics of pleasure: Female sexual appetite in the Hippocratic corpus. *Helios* 19:72-91.

Deane, Paul. 2003. *Sex and the paranormal*. London: Vega.

DeAngelis, Tori. 2003. Considering creativity, dream on. *APA Monitor on Psychology* 34, no. 10: 48. Accessed 25 July 2005 at www.apa.org/monitor/nov03/dreamon.html

Delaney, Gayle. 1994. Sexual dreams: Why we have them, what they mean. New York: Ballantine Books. Retitled as *Sensual dreaming: How to understand and interpret the erotic content of your dreams.*

Dement, W. and N. Kleitman. 1957. Cyclic variations in EEG during sleep and their relation to eye movements, body motility, and dreaming. *Electroencephalography and Clinical Neurophysiology* 9:672-90.

Dement, William C. 1974. *Some must watch while some must sleep.* New York: W.W. Norton and Co., Inc.

------. 1992. *Sleepwatchers.* Stanford, CA: Stanford Alumni Asso.

------. 1999. *Sleep paralysis.* Accessed 22 September 2005 at www.stanford.edu/~dement/paralysis.html

Domhoff, G. William. 2001. Why did empirical dream researchers reject Freud? A critique of historical claims by Mark Solms. *Dreaming* 14:3-17. Updates accessed 21 June 2005 at http://psych.ucsc.edu/dreams/Library/domhoff_2004c.html

------. 1996. *Finding meaning in dreams: A quantitative approach.* New York: Plenum.

DSM-IV. 1994. *Diagnostic and statistical manual of mental disorders.* 4th ed. Washington, D.C.: American Psychiatric Association.

Dutton, D. G. and A. P. Aron. 1974. Some evidence for heightened sexual attraction under conditions of high anxiety. *Journal of Personality and Social Psychology* 30:510-517.

Eagan, John. 2004. Dream lover. *Musclemag.* 275: 246. Accessed 28 February 2005 at www.emusclemag.com/default.asp?pagename=sexmatters&issue=275

Eisler, Riane. 1995. *Sacred pleasure: Sex, myth, and the politics of the body.* San Francisco: Harper.

Elliot, Leland and Cynthia Brantley. 1997. *Sex on campus: The naked truth about the real sex lives of college students.* New York: Random House.

Ellis, Havelock. 1936. [1898]. *Studies in the psychology of sex, vol. I, pt.1.* (Rev. ed). New York: Random House.

Epilepsy Ontario. 2005. *Seizures.* Accessed 17 September 2005 at http://epilepsyontario.org/client/eo/eoweb.nsf

Evans, E. P. 1906. *The criminal prosecution and capital punishment of animals.* London.

Fisher, C, J. Gross, and J. Zuch, 1965. Cycle of penile erections synchronous with dreaming (REM) sleep. *Archives of General Psychiatry* 12:29-45.

Fisher, C., H.D. Cohen, R.C. Schiavi, D. Davis, B. Furman, K. Ward, A. Edwards, and J Cunningham. 1983. Patterns of female sexual arousal during sleep and waking: Vaginal thermo-conductance studies. *Archives of Sexual Behavior* 12, no. 2:97-122.

Fisher, Seymour. 1989. *Sexual images of the self: The psychology of erotic sensations and illusions.* Hillsdale, NJ: Lawrence Erlbaum Associates.

Fisher, S. and R. Greenberg. 1977. *The scientific credibility of Freud's theories and therapy.* New York: Basic Books.

------. 1996. *Freud scientifically appraised.* New York: Wiley.

Finkelstein, Jordan W. et al. 1998. Effects of estrogen or testosterone on self-reported sexual responses and behaviors in hypogonadal adolescents. *Journal of Clinical Endocrinology and Metabolism* 83, no. 7:2281.

Flanagan, Owen. 2000. *Dreaming souls.* New York: Oxford University Press.

Foucault, Michel. 1978. Eng. trans. *The history of sexuality, vol. 1.* New York: Random House.

------. 1985. Eng. trans. *The history of sexuality, vol. 2.* New York: Random House.

Foulkes, D. 1962. Dream reports from different stages of sleep. *Journal of Abnormal and Social Psychology* 65:14-25.

------. 1985. *Dreaming: A cognitive-psychological analysis.* Mahwah, NJ: Erlbaum.

Freud, Sigmund. 1900. *The interpretation of dreams.* In *The basic writings of Sigmund Freud.* 1995. Translated and edited by A. A. Brill. New York: Random House.

------. 1905. *Three contributions to the theory of sex.* In *The basic writings of Sigmund Freud.* 1995. Translated and edited by A. A. Brill. New York: Random House.

Friesen, Wendi. 2003. *Hypnotic ultimate orgasm.* Accessed 10 April 2005 at www.biggerisbetter.com; and www.wendi.com

Gackenbach, J., and J. Bosveld. 1989. *Control your dreams*. New York: Harper and Row.

Gackenbach, J. 1990. Women and meditators as gifted lucid dreamers. In *Dreamtime and Dreamwork*, ed. S. Krippner, 244-51. Los Angeles: Jeremy Tarcher.

Gadon, Elinor W., 1989. *The once and future Goddess*. New York: Harper & Row.

Garfield, Patricia. 1974. *Creative dreaming*. New York: Simon and Schuster.

------. 1979. *Pathway to ecstasy*. New York: Holt, Reinhart & Winston.

Gebhard, P. H., J. Raboch, and H. Geise. 1970. *The sexuality of women*. Bearne, trans. New York: Stein and Day.

Geddes, Donald P. 1954. *An analysis of the Kinsey Reports on sexual behavior in the human male and female*. New York: New American Library.

Goldstein, L., N. W. Stoltzfus, and J. F. Gardocki. 1972. Changes in interhemispheric amplitude relationships in the EEG during sleep. *Physiology and Behaviour* 8:811-15.

Good Vibrations. Accessed 25 March 2005 at www.goodvibrations.com

Good Wife. 2005. *A taste of the Good Wife.* (January 24, 2005). Accessed 25 March 2005 at www.thegoodwife.blogspot.com/2005/01/nocturnal-orgasms.html

Gottesmann, C 1999. Neurophysiological support of consciousness during waking and sleep. *Progress in Neurobiology* 59, no. 5:469-508.

Graham, Janis. 2002. His most secret question. *Redbook*. (May): 43.

Green, C. and C. McCreery. 1994. *Lucid dreaming: The paradox of consciousness during sleep*. London: Routledge.

Guilleminault, C., A. Moscovitch, K. Yuen, and D. Poyares. 2002. Atypical sexual behavior during sleep. *Journal of Psychosomatic Medicine* 64, no. 2:328-36.

Hall, Calvin. 1947. Diagnosing personality by the analysis of dreams. *Journal of Abnormal and Social Psychology* 42:68-79.

------. 1967. Representation of the laboratory setting in dreams. *Journal of Nervous and Mental Disease* 144:198-206.

Hall, Calvin and Robert Van de Castle. 1966. *The content analysis of dreams*. New York: Appleton-Century-Croft.

Hall, Lesley A. 1992. Forbidden by God, despised by men: Masturbation, medical warnings, moral panic, and manhood in Great Britain, 1850-1950. *Journal of the History of Sexuality* 2, no.1. Downloaded 25 May 2005 from: www.highbeam.com

Hamann, Stephan, Rebecca A. Herman, Carla L. Nolan, and Kim Wallen. 2004. Men and women differ in amygdala response to visual sexual stimuli. *Nature Neuroscience* 7: 411-16.

Hartman, William and Marilyn A. Fithian. 1972. *Treatment of sexual dysfunction – A bio-psycho-social approach*. Long Beach, CA: Center for Marital and Sexual Studies.

Hartmann, E. 1966. Dreaming sleep and the menstrual cycle. *Journal of Nervous and Mental Disorders* 143: 406-416.

Heiman, M. 1976. Sleep orgasm in women. *Journal of the American Psychoanalytical Society* 24, no. 5:285-304.

Heiman, Julia, Leslie LoPiccolo, and Joseph LoPiccolo. 1976. *Becoming orgasmic: A sexual growth program for women.* New Jersey: Prentice-Hall.

Henton, C. L. 1976. Nocturnal orgasm in college women: Its relation to dreams and anxiety associated with sexual factors. *The Journal of Genetic Psychology* 129:245-251.

Herman, J., S. El man, and H. Roffwarg. 1978. The problem of NREM dream recall reexamined. in *The Mind In Sleep: Psychology and Psychophysiology.* A. Arkin, J. Antrobus, and S. Ellman, eds., 59-62. Mahwah, New Jersey: Erlbaum.

Hite, Shere. 1976. *The Hite report.* New York: Macmillan Publishing Co.

------. 1994. *The Hite report on the family.* New York: Grove Press.

Hobson, J. A., and R. McCarley. 1977. The brain as a dream state generator: An activation-synthesis hypothesis of the dream process. *American Journal of Psychiatry* 134:1335-1348.

Hobson, J.A. 1988. *The dreaming brain.* New York: Basic Books.

Hobson, J.A., R. Stickgold, E.F. Pace-Schott. 1998. The neuropsychology of REM sleep dreaming. *NeuroReport* 9, no. 3:R1-14.

Hobson, J.A., E.F Pace-Schott, and R. Stickgold. 2000. Dreaming and the brain: Toward a cognitive neuroscience of conscious states. *Behavioral and Brain Sciences* 23: 293-342.

Hoffmann, Heather, Erick Janssen, and Stefanie L. Turner. 2004. Classical conditioning of sexual arousal in women and men: Effects of varying awareness and biological relevance of the conditioned stimulus. *Archives of Sexual Behavior* 33, no. 1:43-53.

Holloway, Gillian. 2001. *The complete dream book: Discover what your dreams tell about you and your life.* Naperville, IL: Sourcebooks.

Holloway, Gillian. 1995-2005. *Dream incubation.* Accessed 12 June 2005 at www.lifetreks.com/lifetreks2/incubation.asp

Holstege, Gert. 2005(a). Human brain imaging of orgasm in males and females. In *Book of Abstracts.* Conference of the International Academy of Sex Research. Ottawa. July 2005.

------. 2005(b). The orgasmic brain. Interview transcript from *All in the Mind.* Australian Broadcasting Corporation, Radio National. July 9, 2005. Accessed 6 September 2005 at www.abc.net.au/rn/science/mind/stories/s1407052.htm

Holstege, Gert, Janniko R. Georgiadis, Anne M. J. Paans, Linda C. Meiners, Ferdinand H.C. E van der Graaf, and A. A. T. Simome Reinders. 2003. Brain activation during human male ejaculation. *Journal of Neuroscience* 23, no. 27:9185-9193.

Holstege, Gert et al., 2005. PET scan results of brain activity during male and female orgasm. Research at Groningen University. Presentation at *European Society of Human Reproduction and Embryology* Conference in Copenhagen. 20 June 2005.

Hoon, P. W., J. P. Wincze, and E. F. Hoon. 1977. A test of reciprocal inhibition: Are anxiety and sexual arousal in women mutually inhibitory? *Journal of Abnormal Psychology* 86:65-74.

Hufford, David J. 1976. A new approach to 'The Old Hag': The nightmare tradition reexamined. In *American Folk Medicine.* W.D. Hand, ed. Los Angeles: University of California Press.

------. 1982. *The terror that comes in the night: An experience-centered study of supernatural assault traditions.* Philadelphia: University of Pennsylvania Press.

------. 2005. Sleep paralysis as spiritual experience. *Transcultural Psychiatry* 42, no. 1:11-45.

Hyde, Deborah. 2005. *Unnatural predators: Vampires and vampyres.* Accessed 12 October 2005 at www.arkanefx.com/unpred/sexpred/incsucc.html

Irvine, Janice M. 1990. *Disorders of desire: Sex and gender in modern American sexology.* Philadelphia: Temple University Press.

Jaccard, R. 1975. *L'exil interieure.* Paris: PUF.

Janszky, J., A. Szucs, P. Halasz, C. Borbely, A. Hollo, P. Barsi, and Z. Mirnics. 2002. Orgasmic aura originates from the right hemisphere. *Neurology* 58:302-04.

Janus, Samuel S., and Cynthia L. Janus. 1993. *The Janus report on sexual behavior.* New York: John Wiley & Sons, Inc.

Jarvis, Marcy. 2003. In your dreams! – Unconscious female orgasms. *Clean Sheets Erotica Magazine.* Accessed 24 February 2005 at www.cleansheets.com/articles/jarvis_06.18.03.shtml

Kaplan, Helen Singer. 1974. *The new sex therapy.* New York: Brunner/Mazel.

Karacan, I. 1970. Clinical value of nocturnal erection in the prognosis and diagnosis of impotence. *Medical Aspects of Human Sexuality* 4:27-34.

Karacan, I., R. Williams, and P. Salis. 1970. The effect of sexual intercourse on sleep pattern and nocturnal penile erections. *Psychophysiology* 7:333.

Karacan, I. et al. 1976. The ontogeny of nocturnal penile tumescence. *Waking and Sleeping* 1:27-44.

Kelsey, M. 1968. *Dreams: The dark speech of the spirit.* New York: Doubleday.

Kempner, Martha. 2003. A controversial decade: 10 years of tracking debates around sexuality. *SIECUS Report.* September 22, 2003. Downloaded 24 April 2005 from High Beam Research. www.highbeam.com

Kinsey, Alfred C., Wardell B. Pomeroy, Clyde E. Martin. 1948. *Sexual behavior in the human male.* Philadelphia: W.B. Saunders Company.

Kinsey, Alfred C., Wardell B. Pomeroy, Clyde E. Martin, and Paul H. Gebhard. 1953. *Sexual behavior in the human female.* Philadelphia: W.B. Saunders Company.

Kinsey Institute. 2005. *Selected research findings from Kinsey's studies.* Accessed 1 March 2005 at www.indiana.edu/~kinsey/resources/ak-data.html

Kramer, H. and J. Sprenger. 1971, [1486]. *Malleus maleficarum.* English translation by M. Summers and J. Rodker, 1928. Reprinted with 1948 introduction in 1971. New York: Dover Publications.

Kramer, Samuel Noah. 1963. *The Sumerians.* Chicago: University of Chicago Press.

Kremsdorf, Ross B., Lucy J. Palladino, Douglas D. Polenz, and Barbara J. Anista. 1978. Effects of the sex of both interviewer and subject on reported manifest dream content. *Journal of Consulting and Clinical Psychology* 46, no. 5:1166-7.

Kuriansky, Judy. 2002. *The complete idiot's guide to Tantric sex*. Indianapolis: Alpha Books.

LaBerge, S., W. Greenleaf, and B. Kedzierski. 1983. Physiological responses to dreamed sexual activity during lucid REM sleep. *Psychophysiology* 20:454-5.

LaBerge, Stephen. 1985. *Lucid dreaming*. New York: Ballantine.

------. 1990. Lucid dreaming: Psychophysiological studies of consciousness during REM sleep. In *Sleep and Cognition*. R.R. Bootzen, J. F. K hlstron, and D. L. Schacter, eds. 1990. 109-126. Washington, D. C.: American Psychological Association.

LaBerge, Stephen, and Howard Rheingold. 1990. *Exploring the world of lucid dreaming*. New York: Ballantine Books.

Ladas, Alice K., Beverly Whipple, and John D. Perry. 1983. *The G spot and other recent discoveries about human sexuality*. New York: Holt, Rinehart and Winston.

Lamberti, Patty. 2005. *Women's top sexual fantasies*. Accessed 10 August 2005 at www.CompuserveMen.com

Lancre, P. de. 1982 [1613]. *Tableau de l'inconstance des mauvais anges et demons*. N. Jacques-Chaquin. ed. Paris: Aubier.

Laumann, E.O., John H. Gagnon, Robert T. Michael, and Stuart Michaels. 1994. *The social organization of sexuality*. Chicago: University of Chicago Press.

Leitenberg, Harold, Detzer, Mark J., and Srebnik, Debra. 1993. Gender differences in masturbation and the relation of masturbation experience in preadolescence and/or early adolescence to sexual behavior and sexual adjustment in young adulthood. *Archives of Sexual Behavior* 22, no. 2: 87-98.

Letourneau, Elizabeth J. and William O'Donohue. 1997. Classical conditioning of female sexual arousal. *Archives of Sexual Behavior* 26, no. 1:63-78.

Levack, B. P. 1992. *The witch-hunt in early modern europe.* Longman Group: UK Limited.

LoPiccolo, Joseph, and Charles Lobitz. 1972. The role of masturbation in the treatment of orgasmic dysfunction. *Archives of Sexual Behavior* 2, no. 2:163-171.

Mah, Kenneth and Yitzchak Binik. 2005. Are orgasms in the mind or the body? Psychosocial versus physiological correlates of orgasmic pleasure and satisfaction. *Journal of Sex and Marital Therapy* 31, no. 3:187-200.

Maltz, Wendy, and Suzie Boss. 2001. *Private thoughts: Exploring the power of women's fantasies.* New York: New World Library.

Mangan, M. A. 2004. A phenomenology of problematic sexual behavior occurring in sleep. *Archives of Sexual Behavior* 33, no. 3:287-93.

------. 2005. *Sexomnia Bulletin – April, 2005*. Accessed 23 June 2005 at www.Sleepsex.org

Martell, Rael. 2003. Things that go off in the night. *Discovery Health*. Accessed 28 February 2005 at www.discoveryhealth.co.uk/general

Maslow, Abraham H. 1942. Self-esteem (dominance-feeling) and sexuality in women. *Journal of Social Psychology* 16: 259-294. Reprinted in DeMartino, M.F. ed., 1963. 113-143. *Sexual behavior and personality characteristics.* New York: Citadel Press.

Masters, R.E.L. 1966. *Eros and evil: The sexual psychopathology of witchcraft.* New York: Matrix House Publishers.

Masters, William H., and Virginia E. Johnson. 1966. *Human sexual response*. Boston: Little, Brown & Co.

------. 1970. *Human sexual inadequacy*. Boston: Little, Brown & Co.

Masters, William H., Virginia E Johnson, Robert C. Kolodny. 1982. *Masters and Johnson on sex and human loving*. Boston: Little Brown & Co.

Meston Cindy M., and Gorzalka Boris B. 1995. The effects of sympathetic activation on physiological and subjective sexual arousal in women. *Behaviour Research and Therapy* 33:651- 664.

------. 1996a. Differential effects of sympathetic activation on sexual arousal in sexually dysfunctional and functional women. *Journal of Abnormal Psychology* 105:582-591.

------. 1996b. The effects of immediate, delayed, and residual sympathetic activation on sexual arousal in women. *Behaviour Research and Therapy* 34:143-148.

Meston, Cindy, and Julia Heiman. 1998. Ephedrine-activated physiological sexual arousal in women. *Archives of General Psychiatry* 55:652-656.

Meston, Cindy, and Penny F. Frohlich. 2003. Love at first fright: Partner salience moderates roller-coaster-induced excitation transfer. *Archives of Sexual Behavior* 32, no. 6:537-544.

Meston, Cindy, Elaine Hull, Roy J. Levin, and Marca Sipski. 2004. Disorders of orgasm in women. *The Journal of Sexual Medicine* 1:66-68.

Miller, Laurence. 1986. In search of the unconscious; evidence for some cornerstones of Freudian theory is coming from an unlikely source – Basic reuroscience. *Psychology Today* 20, no. 12:60.

Michael, Robert T., John H. Gagnon, Edward O. Laumann, and Gina Kolata. 1994. *Sex in America – A definitive survey.* New York: Little, Brown and Company.

Monaghan, Patricia. 1997. *The new book of goddesses and heroines.* New York: Llewellyn.

Morin, Jack. 1995. *The erotic mind.* New York: Harper Collins.

Muzur, A., E.F. Pace-Schott, and J. A. Hobson. 2002. The prefrontal cortex in sleep.
   Trends in Cognitive Science 6, no. 11:475-481.

National Sleep Foundation. 2004. *Women and sleep.* Accessed 5 July 2005 at www.sleepfoundation.org/hottopics/index.php?secid=17&id=163

NINDS (National Institute of Neurological Disorders and Stroke). 2005. NIH Publication No. 04-3440-c. Accessed 12 August 2005 at

www.ninds.nih.gov/disorders/brain_basics/understanding_sleep.ht m

Occhionero, Miranda. 2004. Mental processes and the brain during dreaming. *Dreaming* 14, no. 1:54-64.

Palace, Eileen M., and Boris. B. Gorzalka. 1990. The enhancing effects of anxiety on arousal in sexually dysfunctional and functional women. *Journal of Abnormal Psychology* 99, no. 4:403-11.

Pass, Cleo Massicotte, 1996. Sleep dreams of women in the childbearing years: A review of research. *Holistic Nursing Practice.* (July): 65-77.

Pellauer, Mary D. 1993. The moral significance of female orgasm: Toward sexual ethics that celebrates women's sexuality. In *Sexuality and the sacred. Sources for theological reflection.* Sandra P. Longfellow and James B. Nelson, eds., 149-168. Louisville, KY: Westminster/John Knox Press.

Persinger, Michael. 1987. *Neuropsychological base of God beliefs.* New York: Praeger.

Persinger, Michael. 2000-2005. *Neuroscience Research Group* at Laurentian University, Ontario, Canada. Accessed 19 October 2005 at www.laurentian.ca/neurosci/_people/Persinger.htm

Persona humana. 1975. trans. Paul Halsall. Catholic Library. Accessed 17 October 2005 at www.newadvent.org/library/docs/_df75se.htm

Planned Parenthood. 2005. Accessed 12 April 2005 at www.plannedparenthood.org

Playboy Magazine. 2005. College sex 101. (October): 102-106.

QueenDom 1996-2005. *Previous Sex-A-Polls: Sexual Fantasies.* Accessed 3 September 2005 at www.QueenDom.com

Reich, Wilhelm. 1973 [1942]. *The function of the orgasm.* (Reprint) New York: Simon & Schuster.

Reinisch, June M., with Ruth Beasley. 1990. *The Kinsey Institute new report on sex.* New York: St. Martin's Press.

Rellini, Alessandra, Katie M. McCall, Patrick K. Randall, and Cindy M. Meston. 2005. The relationship between women's subjective and physiological sexual arousal. *Psychophysiology* 42, no. 1:116-124.

Rhawn, Joseph. 1996. Chapter 4. Emotional brain development. *Neuropsychiatry, neuropsychology, clinical neuroscience, 2nd ed.* New York: Lippincott, Willams & Wilkins.

Richardson, Peggy. 1996. Sleep in pregnancy. *Holistic Nursing Practice* (July): 65-77.

Robbins, Paul R., Roland H. Tank, and Faraneh Houshi. 1985. Anxiety and dream symbolism. *Journal of Personality* 53, no. 1:17-22.

Rogers, Gary S., Robert. L. Van de Castle, William S. Evans, and Joseph W. Critelli. 1985. Vaginal pulse amplitude response patterns during erotic conditions and sleep. *Archives of Sexual Behavior* 14, no. 4:327-42.

Rosenfeld, D. S., A. J. Elhajjar. 1998. Sleepsex: A variant of sleepwalking. *Archives of Sexual Behavior* 27, no. 3:269-278.

Ruff, R. L. 1980. Orgasmic epilepsy [letter]. *Neurology* 30, no. 11:1252.

Schredl, M. and F. Hofmann. 2003. Continuity between waking activities and dream activities. *Journal of Conscious Cognition* 12, no. 2:298-308.

Schulz, David A. 1984. *Human sexuality*. Englewood Cliffs, NJ: Prentice Hall.

Sexuality Information and Education Council of the United States (SIECUS). 1996. *Guidelines for comprehensive sexuality education, kindergarten-12th Grade* – 2nd Edition. Accessed 11 May 2005 from High Beam Research www.highbeam.com

Shafik, Ahmed, Olfat El Sibai, Ali Shafik, Ismail Ahmed, and Randa M. Mostafa. 2004. Electrovaginogram: Study of the vaginal electric activity and its role in the sexual act and disorders. *Archive of Gynecology and Obstetrics* 269, no. 4:282-286.

Shapiro, Colin.M., J. Paul. Fedoroff, and Nikola. N. Trajanovic. 1996. Sexual behavior in sleep: A newly described parasomnia. *Sleep Research* 25:367.

Shapiro, Colin. M., Nikola N. Trajanovic, J. Paul Federoff. 2003. Sexsomnia – A new parasomnia? *Canadian Journal of Psychiatry* 48, no. 5:311-17.

Sherfey, Mary Jane. 1972. *The nature and evolution of female sexuality*. New York: Random House.

Singh, D., W. Meyer, R.J. Zambarano, and D.F. Hurlbert. 1998. Frequency and timing of coital orgasm in women desirous of becoming pregnant. *Archives of Sexual Behavior* 27, no. 1:15-29.

Sjoo, Monica, and Barbara Mor. 1987. *The great cosmic mother*. San Francisco: Harper & Row

Solms, Mark. 1997. *The neuropsychology of dreams: A clinico-anatomical study*. Mahwah, NJ: Erlbaum

Stekel, Wilhelm. 1920. *Der telepathische traum*. Berlin: Johannes Baum.

Stewart, Charles. 2002. Erotic dreams and nightmares from antiquity to the present (research). *Journal of the Royal Anthropological Institute*. 8, no. 2:279-309. Downloaded 4 July 2005 from Highbeam Research: 1-43. www.highbeam.com

Stoller, Robert J. 1979. *Sexual excitement: Dynamics of erotic life*. New York: Simon and Schuster.

Sutton, J., C. Rittenhouse, E. Pace-Schott, R. Stickgold, and J. Hobson. 1994. A new approach to dream bizarreness: Graphing continuity and discontinuity of visual attention in narrative reports. *Consciousness and Cognition* 3:61-88.

Sweeney, Kathleen. 1999. Maiden USA: Representing teenage girls in the '90s. *Afterimage* 26, no.1-2: pgs. unknown. Accessed 10 April 2005 at www.questia.com.

Tapia, F., Werboff, J., and Winokur, G. 1958. Recall of some phenomena of sleep: A comparative study of dreams, somnambulism, orgasm, and enuresis in a control and neurotic population. *Journal of Nervous and Mental Disorders* 127:119-23.

Tart C. 1969. *Altered states of consciousness: A book of readings.* New York: Wiley.

Tennov, Dorothy. 1979. *Love and limerence: The experience of being in love.* Chelsea, Michigan: Scarborough House.

Terman, L. M., and M. H. Oden. 1959. *The gifted group at mid-life.* Stanford, California: Stanford University Press.

Tiefer, Leonore. 1995. *Sex is not a natural act and other essays.* Boulder, CO: Westview Press.

Tissot, Samuel A. 1758 (Latin), 1832 (English). 1974. A treatise on the diseases produced by Onanism. In *The secret vice exposed! Some arguments against masturbation.* Charles Rosenberg and Carroll Smith-Rosenberg, eds., 59-87. New York: ARNO Press.

Ullman, M., S. Krippner, and A. Vaughan. 1973. *Dream telepathy.* New York: Macmillan.

Van de Castle, Robert. 1971. *The psychology of dreaming.* Morristown, N.J: General Learning Press.

-------. 1994. *Our dreaming mind.* New York: Ballantine Books.

Wade, Jenny. 2004. *Transcendent sex.* New York: Simon & Schuster.

Wagner, G. (Producer). 1973. *Physiological responses of the sexually stimulated female in the laboratory* (Film). New York: Focus International.

Weingarten, Toni. 2005. Sacred fire. *Spirituality and Health* 8, no. 2:60-69.

Weisz, R. and D. Foulkes. 1970. Home and laboratory dreams collected under uniform sampling conditions. *Psychophysiology* 6:588-96.

Wells, Barbara L. 1983. Nocturnal orgasms: Females' perceptions of a "normal" sexual experience. *Journal of Sex Education and Therapy* 9:32-38.

-------. 1986. Predictors of female nocturnal orgasms: A multivariate analysis. *Journal*
      of Sex Research 22:421-37.

Weston, Louanr e C. 2005. Can women have wet dreams? *WebMD*. Accessed 28 February 2005 at http://my.webmd.com/content/article/99/105310.htm

Whalen, P.J. 1998. Fear, vigilance, and ambiguity: Initial neuroimaging studies of the human amygdala. *Current Directions in Psychological Science* 7:177-88.

Whipple, Beverly, Gina Ogden, and Barry R. Komisaruk. 1992. Physiological correlates of imagery-induced orgasm in women. *Archives of Sexual Behavior* 21, no. 2:121-33.

Whipple, Beverly, and Barry R. Komisaruk. 1985. Elevation of pain threshold by vaginal stimulation in women. *Pain* 21:357-67.

-------. 1988. Analgesia produced in women by genital self-stimulation. *Journal of Sex Research* 24:130-40.

Wiley, Diana. 2005. Product endorsement for natural contours. Accessed 2 March 2005 at http://www.natural-contours.com/Endorse.asp?cookie%5Ftest=1

Winokur, G., Guze, S. B., and Pfeiffer, A. B. 1959. Nocturnal orgasm in women: Its relation to psychiatric illness, dreams and developmental and sexual factors. *A.M.A. Archives of General Psychiatry* 1:180-84.

Wong, Mildred. 2002. Because it's there: Morals, medicine and masturbation in the nineteenth century. *University of Toronto Medical Journal* 79, no. 3:263-65.

Zillman, D. 1971. Excitation transfer in communication mediated aggressive behavior. *Journal of Experimental Social Psychology* 7:419-434.

Zohar (3:76). in Patai, R. 1981. *Gates to the old city*. Detroit: Wayne State University.

www.ingramcontent.com/pod-product-compliance
Lightning Source LLC
Chambersburg PA
CBHW060244290526
45789CB00001B/193